THE
GOOD DOCTOR'S GUIDE
TO COLDS AND FLU

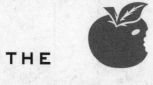

Neil Schachter, M.D.

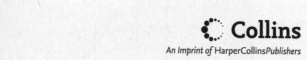

Collins
An Imprint of HarperCollinsPublishers

HarperCollins books may be purchased for educational, business, or sales
promotional use. For information, please write: Special Markets Department,
HarperCollins Publishers, 10 East 53rd Street, New York, NY 10022.

FIRST EDITION 2005

Designed by Nicola Ferguson

Illustrations by Eric Faltreco

Library of Congress Cataloging-in-Publication Data

Schachter, Neil.
    The good doctor's guide to colds and flu / Neil Schachter.
        p.   cm.
    Includes index.
    ISBN-10: 0-06-076249-7
    ISBN-13: 978-0-06-076249-0
    1. Cold (Disease)—Popular works.   2. Influenza—Popular works.
3. Respiratory infections—Popular works.   I. Title.

RF361.S29   2005
616.2'05—dc22

                                                        2005046233

05   06   07   08   09   WBC/RRD   10   9   8   7   6   5   4   3   2   1

For Deborah,

You have done so much for all of us. You are the glue, the strength and resolve that has held us together as well as the vision that kept us moving forward.

ACKNOWLEDGMENTS

I would like to acknowledge the support and friendship of: My colleagues at Mount Sinai: Drs. Mike Iannuzzi, Meyer Kattan, Alvin Tierstein, Gwen Skloot, David Nierman, Maria Padilla, Phillip Landrigan, Eugenia Zuskin, Judith Nelson, Tom Kalb, Scott Lorin, Cynthia Caracta, Sharon Camhi, Michelle Gong, David Kaufman, Juan Wisnivesky, Lori Shah, and Stasia Wieber. Special thanks to Kay Derman of the Mount Sinai Volunteer Department, who has provided me the opportunity to work with young doctors-to-be in my laboratory.

The staff and board members of the American Lung Association of the City of New York—Louise Vetter; my friend and mentor Robert Mellins, M.D.; Peter Smith, M.D.; Bernadette Murphy; Rob Roth; Neil Schluger, M.D.; David Rappaport, M.D.; Joan Reibman, M.D.; Lester Blair, M.D.; and Rami Bachiman.

The incredible staff at Mount Sinai: My friend and right arm Teo Hoke, Judith Schneiderman, Angelo Chiarelli, Katherine Barboza, Lourdes Mateo, Michelle Solomon, Rachel Posner, and Shirly Palleja. Thanks go to Ian Ochshorn, Joe Widowski, and the staff of the Respiratory Care Department who work tirelessly to provide caring and critical services to our sickest patients.

My colleagues from Yale University: Drs. Herbert Reynolds; Arend Bouhuys (the late chief of Pulmonary Medicine); Arthur Dubois of the Pierce Foundation at Yale; Michael Littner; Theodore Witek, now with Boehringer Ingelheim; Michael Niederman, now chief of Pulmonary Medicine at Winthrop University Hospital; Richard Matthay, Vice Chair of Medicine at Yale University School of Medicine; and Samuel O. Thier, former chief of Medicine at Yale.

My colleagues on the frontline of COPD: John Walsh, CEO of the COPD Foundation; Sam Giordano, CEO of the AARC; Claude Lenfant, former chief of the NHLBI; Shri Nair, M.D., of Yale Norwalk; Bart Celli, M.D., of Tufts University; Barbara Rogers of NECA; Linda Marshall of the American Legacy Foundation; Barry Make, M.D., of the National Jewish Hospital in Denver; Robert Sandhaus, M.D., of Alpha-1 Foundation; and William Kutscher of the Emphysema/COPD *Journal of Patient Centered Care.*

My fellow soldiers in the battle with the tobacco industry and environmental health: Joe Cherner, founder of Smoke Free Educational Services; Hurbert Humphrey III, former governor of Minnesota; Ira Burnim of the Southern Poverty Law Office; and Eric Frumin of ACTWU.

My artist, Eric Faltreco, for the beautiful illustrations and web design; Denise Mann for her timely editorial assistance; and to my agent, Marly Rusoff, for her continual support.

My fellow pulmonologists: Peter Barnes of the National Heart and Lung Institute in London; Nicholas Gross, M.D., of the Stritch School of Medicine of Loyola University; Dean Hess, RRT, of Massachusetts General Hospital; and Neil MacIntyre, M.D., of Duke University.

My teachers and colleagues at NYU Medical Center: The late John McClement, M.D.; Saul Farber, M.D.; Martin Kahn, M.D.; Arthur Localio, M.D.; and Joseph Ransohoff, M.D.

To Alfred La Spina of Kaz/Honeywell, who provided invaluable support to education programs for better pulmonary health; to Rachel Littner whose PR expertise created "buzz."

The staff at HarperCollins: My wise and very patient editor, Toni Sciarra, who made this book a pleasure to write; Shelby Meizlik in publicity; and Collins U.S. president, Joe Tessitore, whose well-crafted suggestions gave the book the personal touch it needed.

CONTENTS

CHAPTER 1: WELCOME TO THE COLD WARS, *1*

CHAPTER 2: THE SCENE OF THE CRIME, *11*

CHAPTER 3: TREATMENT—THE RIGHT CHOICE AT THE RIGHT TIME, *27*

CHAPTER 4: COLDS 101, *59*

CHAPTER 5: SINUSITIS—THE COLD THAT LINGERS, *74*

CHAPTER 6: BRONCHITIS—WHEN A COUGH IS MORE THAN A COUGH, *94*

CHAPTER 7: STREP THROAT—WHEN IT EVEN HURTS TO SWALLOW, *117*

CHAPTER 8: PNEUMONIA—WHEN A COLD TURNS SERIOUS, *127*

CHAPTER 9: INFLUENZA—THE COLD'S EVIL TWIN, *153*

CHAPTER 10: THE SNEEZING YEARS—COLDS AND FLU IN CHILDHOOD, *175*

CHAPTER 11: INDIVIDUAL NEEDS, INDIVIDUAL
            SOLUTIONS, 197

CHAPTER 12: COMMON QUESTIONS AND ANSWERS, 216

INDEX, 233

CHAPTER 1

WELCOME TO
THE COLD WARS

There are three things that I know about Katherine Davis. She is the author of twenty-two romance novels, stands six feet tall in her stockinged feet, and she never, ever calls me unless something is seriously wrong.

I first met Katherine when her husband was hit by a mini-van. As he was brought to the emergency room, his lung collapsed and I was called for a consultation. While we were working on Nate, his heart stopped briefly and we had to scramble to get his cardiac system working again. The next time Katherine called, her furnace had had a puff back and she and her family had inhaled oily, black soot. So when she called me again at home late on a rainy spring night, I imagined the worst.

"Neil, I can't believe what happened!" she began anxiously.

I peppered her with questions: "Is Nate all right? Is he short of breath? Is he in pain?"

"No! No!" she exclaimed. "It's this awful cold! You doctors can bring people back from the dead. Isn't there anything that you can do for this miserable stuffed nose and sore throat?"

I was so relieved that I burst out laughing. "It's not funny!" she wailed. "We had to cancel our trip to Italy because of this stupid cold."

Katherine is hardly unique in her cold or in her sense of frustration. Each year Americans suffer an astonishing 1 billion colds. We spend $5 billion on cold and sniffle remedies. These all-too-common virus infections are responsible for the loss of 50 million workdays and 60 million school days. Influenza, the simple cold's evil twin, affects up to 60 million Americans and is fatal to twenty thousand people annually. In fact, influenza and pneumonia together are the sixth leading cause of death in the United States.

The Good Doctor's Guide to Colds and Flu will show you how to avoid illness, the most effective approachs to reducing congestion, fever, and discomfort when a cold, flu, or other respiratory infections do strike, and what to do if an infection becomes serious.

We tend to call any illness accompanied by coughs and sneezes a cold, but there are actually six different types of respiratory infections that begin with seemingly similar symptoms. In addition to colds and flu, bronchitis, pneumonia, sore throats, and sinusitis affect different parts of the respiratory system and require individualized strategies for prevention and treatment. For example, Katherine Davis's cold had actually developed into bronchitis, and she needed a short course of bronchodilators to reduce irritability of her airways. If her cold had been treated early and correctly, she could likely have avoided the lung problems that forced cancellation of her trip.

While modern diseases such as SARS and mad cow disease have captured the world's attention, the history of colds is as old as the history of man. Early Egyptian hieroglyphs depicting cough and cold are found on the walls of ancient buildings. The famous Ebers papyrus offered a potion for cold symptoms called galena that included dry incense and honey. The earliest description of a cold was given by fifth-century B.C. Greek physician Hippocrates, who is considered the father of medicine. Hippocrates carefully described a runny, swollen nose and fever. He did not offer remedies, but he rightly rejected his era's favored approach of bleeding as a cure for colds.

The care of colds, considered a minor problem, was left to homemade concoctions and folk medicine, a tradition that continues today. In the first century, Pliny the Elder recommended kissing the hairy muzzle of a mouse for the relief of cold symptoms. At that same period of time in Rome, Celsus wrote about the common cold and prescribed a more popular remedy—flagons of good Italian wine. Wine, warm and spiced, has reappeared as a cold remedy over the centuries and is still used today.

During the fifteenth and sixteenth centuries, hot drinks that raised a sweat were thought to be the perfect antidote for the cold. Ben Franklin declared that fresh air prevented colds, since he observed that colds were contracted by close contact with other cold sufferers. He was also probably the first who dismissed the idea that cold or dampness produced this illness.

Over the centuries the cause of colds and sniffles remained even more elusive. The Greeks thought the symptoms were due to an imbalance of humors, while the Saxons were convinced the disease was due to invisible arrows flying through the air. Among Pueblo Indians, respiratory diseases were thought to be due to serpents and spirits and demons entering the body. The solution was a ceremony in which disease witches were whipped away with eagle plumes.

In the latter half of the nineteenth century, a brilliant French chemist named Louis Pasteur and a dedicated German physician named Robert Koch made a series of discoveries that ushered in the golden age of microbiology. Pasteur, Koch, and the students they trained systematically isolated and identified the causes of the major killer diseases. Typhus, typhoid fever, tuberculosis, syphilis, and even leprosy were no longer mysteries—but the cause of the common cold was still unknown. It took two world wars and a cataclysmic influenza pandemic for scientists in England and the United States to persuade officials of the need to study these widespread ailments.

Their commitment led to the creation of the Common Cold Unit, located in a remote corner of England near Salisbury. The goals of this unit were both simple and ambitious: to discover the causes of colds, understand their transmission, and develop vaccines and cures.

Over the next fifty years, the scientists of the unit along with their human volunteers identified eight categories of colds and isolated over two hundred different types of viruses. They learned how colds were spread, why stress can affect immunity, and identified links between weather and infection. But both the vaccine and the cure they sought eluded them, and in 1996 the Common Cold Unit was disbanded.

Influenza, the cold's evil twin, has an equally long and interesting history. The term *influenza* was first applied to the disease during an epidemic that occurred in Florence in 1580. The name is an Italian word meaning "influence," a referral to the deleterious influence of the stars on the welfare of humans. Writing in 1659 regarding a widespread illness, Dr. Thomas Wyle described a troublesome cough, a feverish distemper, and a grievous pain in the back and limbs. The seventeenth-century physician, like most medical experts of his era, blamed "the blast of stars" for the illness.

Several hundred years later when medical researchers realized that a virus caused this illness in people, the influenza virus was one of the first viruses that was isolated and grown in a laboratory. For centuries there have been reported influenza outbreaks that have varied in severity and spread. But far more virulent diseases monopolized the attention of doctors and scientists. Compared to bubonic plague, cholera, malaria, and typhoid fever, influenza was not considered that serious.

Not until the influenza pandemic of 1918–19 were the dangers of the flu virus truly recognized. Half a million Americans died as the result of this epidemic, and as many as 50 million have been estimated to have perished worldwide. The death and destruction wrought by this seemingly routine infection spurred the establishment of virus surveillance and flu vaccine programs. Seen against the impact of such problems as plague, typhoid, smallpox, or malaria, respiratory infections such as colds and flu do seem to be unimportant, but with major epidemics of other infectious diseases now under control, we recognize the importance and nuisance of these all-too-common problems.

With influenza, it is the quantity rather than the quality of this disease that makes it an important public health issue. Government health officials, seeing the impact of influenza outbreaks in lost school days, lost days from work, and lowered productivity, have supported public health outreach and research.

In this society, where we want to take advantage of every opportunity to work and play, coughs, flu, and sneezes are unwelcome intruders. *The Good Doctor's Guide to Colds and Flu* will provide all the latest and most effective information on preventing and relieving respiratory problems. For most people, these illnesses are nuisance problems, but for people with underlying health issues such as asthma, heart disease, and diabetes, these minor illnesses and their treatments present new challenges.

Colds, flus, and other infectious diseases that affect the respiratory system do not get the attention they deserve from the medical community. When coughs and sneezes appear, people are too often left on their own to deal with the symptoms. It's unfortunate because there are safe and effective ways to prevent illness and relieve discomfort, but most people are not given treatment plans. *The Good Doctor's Guide to Colds and Flu* explains the science behind common respiratory infections so that people can successfully manage these routine but frustrating illnesses.

The medical advice for the six key respiratory illnesses are geared for healthy adults. For children and those with underlying health problems, the issues can be different, and separate chapters will point out differences in the course of disease and its treatment in these populations.

Chapter 2, "The Scene of the Crime," familiarizes you with the function of the upper airways, consisting of the nose, sinuses, ears, and throat, and the lower airways, formed by the lungs and the bronchi. It will illustrate the connections between the different parts of the respiratory system and explain how each is affected by colds and viruses that cause illness in the respiratory tract.

I have found that when patients understand how their respiratory system functions, they are better able to understand how to control and prevent these widespread health problems. For example, Nancy Rodriguez, a pack-a-day smoker, came to me because she kept getting colds. She was getting married the next month and was worried that she would walk down the aisle coughing, with a red, runny nose and a sore throat. I explained that the body's first line of defense against colds were cilia in the nose, tiny hairlike structures that sweep viruses, bacteria, and other organisms out of the nose. Unfortunately, cigarette smoking paralyzes cilia, allowing viruses and bacteria to easily enter the respiratory tract. When she realized that her pack-a-day habit had lowered her immunity and caused endless sniffles, she was so tired of watery, red eyes and a lingering cough that she was motivated to quit smoking, albeit just for the wedding.

Chapter 3, "Treatment—the Right Choice at the Right Time," focuses on the medical choices that can prevent disease and relieve symptoms if illness does strike. There is no shortage of effective and/or unusual advice offered for colds and flu. William Osler, the noted nineteenth-century physician, recommended that one place a top hat on a bedpost, get into bed, and keep drinking whiskey until there was a hat on both bedposts.

While the whiskey cure will always have its supporters, a more modern approach focuses on both the inflammation of a cold as well as the replication of viruses.

There are ten different categories of therapies that singly or in combination can help you stay healthier and feel better. For example, the ache and fever of a cold are caused by the release of inflammatory chemicals called cytokines from cells under a viral attack. Aspirin and ibuprofen block the generation of these cytokines, reducing the inflammation and keeping pain and fever under control. Chapter 3 will explain how each type of remedy works, how and when they should be used, and describes potential side effects as well as the best choices for each situation.

Chapter 4, "Colds 101," will explore the signs and symptoms of the all-too-common cold. You'll learn about the different kinds of cold viruses. I'll explain how to know if it's a cold or allergy, why we get more colds in winter, and how to decrease your risk of catching a cold. For example, an important way to lower the risk of our catching a cold is to avoid borrowing a pen. Another even simpler trick is to wash your hands several times a day with soap and water. Viruses can live for hours on inert objects, and pens can be passed to dozens of people in just a few hours of communal use.

Sinus problems affect 37 million Americans each year, and they don't arrive unannounced. Chapter 5, "Sinusitis—the Cold That Lingers," explains how sinusitis often follows a cold or flu. It looks at both acute and chronic sinusitis and explores the symptoms, treatment, and prevention strategies. Chapter 5 examines diagnostic tools for sinus problems such as CT scans, the value of anti-inflammatory treatment, and explores the pros and cons of sinus surgery. This chapter closes with simple tips to prevent sinusitis, including why humming five seconds a day may reduce risk of sinus problems.

Bronchitis is a stalker appearing after a cold or flu. A cold should be over and gone in five to seven days. A cough that develops in the course of a cold and shows no sign of going away is a good indication that bronchitis is now a problem. This type of exhausting cough interrupts sleep and is one of the key symptoms that forces even the busiest person to make time for a visit to the doctor. Chapter 6, "Bronchitis—When a Cough Is More Than a Cough," starts with a look at the changes that occur in the lungs during an episode of bronchitis and continues with an explanation of symptoms, pointing out the differences between acute and chronic bronchitis, as well as other conditions such as asthma, pneumonia, and pleurisy. Chapter 6 closes with the safest and most effective way to prevent developing bronchitis.

Americans make 18 million visits each year to the doctor for painful sore throat known to doctors as pharyngitis. They often call these infections strep throats. Actually, many other organisms produce the same symptoms, including viruses, mycoplasma, and chlamydia. Chapter 7, "Strep Throat—When It Even Hurts to Swallow," looks at the use of throat cultures and immunoassay to identify the cause of symptoms, addresses the risk of heart and kidney disease in strep infections, and reveals a key sign that can differentiate between tonsillitis and a viral sore throat. Chapter 7 closes with a look at the carrier state (persons who are "colonized" with the bacterium but who have no symptoms) versus acute strep throat and how antibiotics can be used to stop the spread of this infection to the rest of the family.

There are respiratory infections and then there is pneumonia. While colds and sore throats can be inconvenient and uncomfortable, pneumonia is actually the sixth leading cause of death in the United States. An estimated 3–4 million cases occur each year, and 1 million people are hospitalized with this serious lung problem. Chapter 8, "Pneumonia—When a Cold Turns Serious," begins with a look at the unique symptoms that are characteristic of pneumonia, the different types of pneumonia, and the prevention techniques that can cut your risk of developing pneumonia. It continues with a look at the differences between bronchial, lobar, and interstitial pneumonia and discusses when pneumonia calls for hospitalization.

Chapter 9, "Influenza—the Cold's Evil Twin," describes the constant variations in influenza viruses, how these viruses damage the respiratory tract, and the best ways to prevent infection. Many people have heard of the flu shot, but they are less aware of oral or inhaled antiviral medications that can prevent or reduce the severity of the flu. Studies have shown that up to 90 percent of people with influenza develop complications of acute bronchitis, and that they may require additional medical intervention to reduce irritability in the airways.

Chapter 10, "The Sneezing Years—Colds and Flu in Childhood," deals with colds and flu in children. All of the recommendations elsewhere in this book are intended for healthy adults, but children are not small adults; they have different immune systems and a different configuration of their respiratory system that need to be taken into account when looking at the causes, prevention, and especially treatment of respiratory infections. This chapter, while certainly not a complete look at respiratory infections in children, will help parents to prevent and treat these illnesses in children from birth through adolescence.

Health issues such as asthma, pregnancy, high blood pressure, diabetes, even advanced age, can make respiratory infections more complicated and dangerous. Chapter 11, "Individual Needs, Individual Solutions," explores the impact of existing health issues on the standard approach to prevention and treatment of respiratory infections. Some conditions, such as asthma, can increase the severity of respiratory problems. In addition, decongestants that relieve the pain and stuffiness of a cold can raise blood pressure, certainly a potential problem if hypertension is already present. Chapter 11 will look at these important differences in symptoms, complications, and treatment of colds, flu, and other common respiratory ailments.

The Good Doctor's Guide to Colds and Flu closes with a question-and-answer section that draws on patients' common questions and my twenty-five years of experience in chest medicine. From questions about the value of wearing a mask to ward off colds and flu to the surprising reason why women catch more colds, chapter 12 will take a sensitive look at the important questions patients have about these all-too-common problems.

THE SCENE
OF THE CRIME

If you read the *Wall Street Journal,* then you know Jack Friedman. Today he sat in my office, staring at me with the same intense blue eyes that for more than thirty years had intimidated bankers on five continents. "Bacteria or virus, I don't care. I just want an antibiotic for this sore throat."

Jack's physician was away, and he had come to me to give him the antibiotics that he took for every sneeze or cough he experienced. Upon examination, it was clear that Jack had a head cold. Looking at his record, I was concerned that when Jack did actually develop a bacterial infection, the bacteria that populate his upper airways would have built up considerable resistance to antibiotics and the medications would no longer work. I picked up a piece of chalk and walked to the small blackboard on the side wall. It was important that Jack understand what was causing his symptoms and why antibiotics were a bad choice. I knew that if I didn't explain why it was not in his best interest to give him what he wanted, he would find another doctor who would.

For the next twenty minutes, I gave Jack a minicourse in his own airways as well as a tip sheet on the bacteria and viruses that cause illness in his nose, throat, and lungs. Jack's eyes drilled into me as I talked. He asked questions, lots of them. Halfway through my impromptu lecture, I could feel the tension level drop in the room. When we finished, Jack agreed to a long-overdue vaccination for pneumonia. For the past five years he had refused to take this lifesaving injection, but when he understood how and why pneumonia is such a serious illness, he asked for it himself.

The great majority of colds and flus are handled without ever consulting a doctor. To relieve symptoms and feel better quickly, it is nevertheless essential to understand both the parts of the body that are affected and the viruses and bacteria that are causing disease and discomfort. You also need to understand what is going on so as to know when it is time to call your physician.

The airways are divided into two sections—the upper and the lower airways. The upper airway starts at the nose, and the architecture of this structure is both complex and efficient. In a small space, the nose performs a number of essential services for the body, and given the small space, it is no surprise that small problems can cause big symptoms.

The interior of the nose is divided into two chambers by a partition called the *nasal septum* (see Illustration on page 13). The division is never perfectly even. One side is always slightly smaller, and this makes it vulnerable to congestion. Protruding from the outer walls of each side of the nasal passageways, called chambers, are three curled plates of bones. These plates are called *turbinates,* and they dramatically increase the surface area inside the nose. The turbinates and the upper airway system are covered by a mucous membrane. This moist surface consists of cells that produce up to two cups of fluid a day called mucus. Mucus maintains a healthy water balance in the nose and acts as a protective coating for all the structures of the nose, helping protect against infection and allergens.

A forest of microscopic, rapidly moving hairs, called *cilia,* propel this mucus into the back of the throat and into the stom-

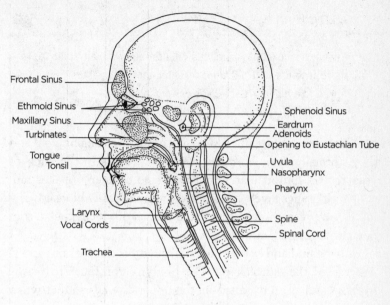

Frontal Sinus

Ethmoid Sinus

Maxillary Sinus

Turbinates

Tongue

Tonsil

Larynx

Vocal Cords

Trachea

Sphenoid Sinus

Eardrum

Adenoids

Opening to Eustachian Tube

Uvula

Nasopharynx

Pharynx

Spine

Spinal Cord

UPPER AIRWAYS

ach, where it is destroyed by digestive fluids. Interestingly, cold viruses paralyze the cilia, inhibiting their ability to clear the airways. The mucus begins to accumulate and harden, leading to a feeling of congestion.

These mucous membranes also contain nerve fibers that are responsible for the sense of smell. When the nose is congested and inflamed, the nerve cells don't function properly, limiting your ability to taste and smell.

Inside the skull there are four groups of sinus cavities. These hollow structures within the bones of the face and skull are somewhat of a mystery. We know that as bony structures, they offer protection to the soft tissues, but we don't really understand their function. It has been suggested that the hollow bones make the skull lighter, and thus it's easier for us to walk upright and support the weight of our head. What we do know for certain is that sinus cavities cause significant health problems.

QUICK TIP

Cigarette smoke also paralyzes cilia, inhibiting their ability to remove irritants and bacteria, a factor that researchers believe is
linked to a higher risk of colds and flu in smokers.

The sinus cavities are lined with mucous membranes, and
they normally drain through two small canals in the back of
your throat. Unfortunately, when a cold or allergy makes mucous membranes swell, the sinus drainage is easily blocked. The
increased pressure of accumulated mucus produces the all-too-
familiar facial pain and headache.

Just behind and below the nasal cavity is the part of the airway called the *nasopharynx*. The pharynx continues to warm,
hydrate, and clean the air from the upper airways so that when
it reaches the lungs, it will be moist and at body temperature.
This five-inch passageway sends air into the lungs and directs
food, water, and mucus to the stomach. When you "swallow
the wrong way," food or liquid gets detoured on its way to the
stomach and winds up in the airways. Your choking and coughing are signs that the body is rerouting these substances out of
the airways.

At the back of the nose and throat are two sometimes troublesome organs: the tonsils and the adenoids. While the main
job of these structures is to provide immune defense, the real
role of these organs seems to be to get infected with bacteria
and viruses. The tonsils, small, spongy patches on either side of
the throat, grow to full size during childhood. At age fifteen,
they start to shrink and almost disappear in adulthood. For
many years, doctors believed that tonsils were the major cause
of childhood respiratory illnesses, and they were routinely removed by the age of six. We now recognize that tonsils actually store white blood cells and, in fact, offer protection against
bacteria and viral infections. Currently, tonsils are only re-

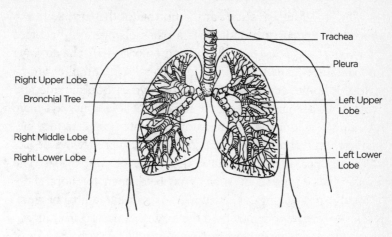

Right Upper Lobe

Bronchial Tree

Right Middle Lobe

Right Lower Lobe

Trachea

Pleura

Left Upper Lobe

Left Lower Lobe

THE LUNGS

moved if they become abnormally large or are continually infected.

Adenoids are a collection of lymphoid tissue (similar to that found in the "glands" that sometimes swell on the neck with a sore throat) near the tonsils. They are located on the back of the throat where the nasal passage connects with the throat. In theory, the adenoids help the body fight off infection, but their main activity seems to be to become enlarged during repeated respiratory infections.

Neighbors of the adenoids, the eustachian tubes lead from the upper throat to each ear. They are designed to drain mucus and keep pressure on the outside of the eardrum equal to that within the semi-enclosed middle ear. A cold or infection can spread up the eustachian tubes and cause earaches, particularly in children.

The upper airways continue into the *larynx* or voice box. Two cordlike structures extend across the larynx to produce your voice. The same type of mucous membrane we have in the nose extends to the walls of the larynx. During a cold or flu, inflammation of this membrane causes hoarseness or even loss of your voice.

The lower airways start at the bottom of the larynx, where the tubelike structure undergoes a name change and becomes known as the *trachea* (see Illustration on page 15). The airways and the lungs have three basic jobs: to take in and filter air, to help the body get oxygen, and to remove carbon dioxide and wastes. To accomplish these three jobs, the lower airways have a beautifully complex organization that interconnects in a mechanical marvel of design. The job of the lower airways begins at the trachea, the large tube in the center of your throat. The trachea is composed of soft tissue held open by horseshoe-shaped cartilage rings. This support is soft enough to be flexible, but strong enough to hold the airways open so that air can pass through. The lower airways continue through the top of the chest, then into and halfway down the breastbone. At this point, the trachea bisects and changes its name. The divisions are now known collectively as the *bronchi*. The right main-stem bronchus leads into your right lung, and the left main-stem bronchus goes into your left lung.

Each lung is divided into lobes, with three on the right side, and two on the left. Each lobe is separated anatomically by a tissue coating called the pleura. It's easy to forget that the pleura plays a role in breathing until it becomes irritated or infected. The irritation causes pain that persists when you're sitting or lying down, and the pain becomes worse when you talk, take a deep breath, or walk.

The bronchi continue to divide within the lobes. When you consider each division as a level, then the bronchial tree, as it is known, divides on average twenty-three times. When you get to those final divisions, you're talking about millions and millions of very, very small airways. It is these airways that become inflamed and swollen when we develop respiratory infections such as pneumonia and bronchitis.

At about the seventeenth division of the bronchi, small sacs called *alveoli* are found surrounding the airways. Each alveolus is basically one cell thick. This is where oxygen enters the

bloodstream and carbon dioxide is removed. In severe infections, the alveoli become damaged, particularly if you've been a
smoker. Smoking damages the alveoli, changing their structure
from neat little balls of grapes to ragged, swollen structures that
can no longer help oxygenate the body. During a cold or flu,
these structures become inflamed. In fact, after a severe lower-
respiratory infection, they can be permanently damaged, leading to a permanently lowered pulmonary function.

The large airways of the pulmonary system are all covered
with a mucous membrane (very much like the membrane that
lines the upper airways), and they also contain mucus-
producing cells, and cilia. In addition, this tissue contains blood
vessels, collagen, and smooth muscles that allow the airways to
contract or relax. When histamine, an irritating body chemical,
is produced, either as a result of an allergy or from infection,
the airways can fill with mucus, and the muscles tighten, narrowing the air passages. In people with asthma, the airway muscles are extremely sensitive, and even minor irritants, such as
cold air or strong smells, can provoke them to narrow the passages, causing difficulty in breathing.

The structures of the airways are the first half of the story
of colds and flus. The second partner in respiratory infections
are the organisms that cause illness.

KNOW YOUR ENEMY

Bacteria and viruses were among the first living organisms on
earth, and long after humans have disappeared as a species, bacteria and viruses will still be living on this planet.

There are over twenty-seven distinct groups of bacteria, and
as many as one hundred strains have been identified in each
group. Bacteria are often beneficial. Without bacteria to break
down dead plants and animals, for example, the earth would be
buried in garbage. Without the right kind of microbes we would

not have good cheese or aged wine. In fact this coexistence is the basis for successful life on earth. Some bacteria attack only plants, while others infect only animals. What concerns us the most are the bacteria and viruses that cause disease in humans.

Bacteria are single-celled organisms that reproduce by dividing. They can live happily outside living cells, but sometimes attach themselves to the membranes of a cell, which interferes with normal cellular activity. The presence of bacteria that are not constrained by normal control systems provokes the body's immune system to release white blood cells and inflammatory compounds such as interleukins and cytokines to defend us. Both of these protective mechanisms produce distinctive symptoms, such as fever, congestion, and fatigue. In addition, bacteria themselves can release toxins that cause similar discomfort.

With thousands of different bacteria in the air and water, doctors have established a number of ways to categorize bacteria and arrive at the best ways to combat them when illness occurs. One of the earliest and still one of the most important methods is to test a bacterium's reaction to a dye used to stain them for recognition under a microscope. Called Gram's stain, this test was developed in 1884 and is still used in every bacteriology lab today. Gram's stain floods a slide covered with infected material with a purple dye, which is then washed off with an acid bath. A second dye is added to color those bacteria that do not "hold" the gram stain. When examined under a microscope, the bacteria that appear purple are called gram-positive. Illnesses that are caused by gram-positive bacteria include strep throat and staph pneumonia. Those that look red are considered gram-negative. Gram-negative organisms have a second membrane or coating that protects them from antibacterial agents such as disinfectants and antibiotics. Not surprisingly, many gram-negative organisms cause serious forms of illness. An example of a gram-negative bacterium is pseudomonas, which can cause an often fatal pneumonia.

We designate bacteria that cause disease in people as *pathogenic*, and those that don't harm us as *nonpathogenic*. When an organism is described as a pathogen, it simply means that it causes disease, not that it causes mild or serious disease. A bacteria that normally lives in our body is called *endogenous*. If it is something we pick up from the environment or from food or from another person, we call it an *exogenous* bacteria—one that comes from the outside.

The oxygen requirements of a bacteria constitute another important way to classify organisms. Bacteria that require the presence of oxygen are called *aerobic*. Those organisms that can only tolerate low levels or no oxygen are known as *anaerobes*. Anaerobes exist harmlessly on the surface of the skin and mucus membranes. If these tissues are injured, anaerobic bacteria can burrow deep into the wound where oxygen levels are low, causing severe, hard-to-treat infections.

Once they enter the body, different bacteria tend to focus on different parts of the body. In this book we are concerned about the health of the airways. Out of the twenty-seven different groups of bacteria that cause disease in humans, only eight cause disease in the nose, throat, or lungs. That's the good news. The bad news is that there are a number of fierce organisms in these eight groups:

1. Staphylococcus aureus (Staph)

We have identified more than thirty different types of these gram-positive organisms that grow in grapelike clusters. These bacteria popularly known as staph commonly live in the nose and throat, and they are a major cause of often serious disease in humans. Some of the most troubling forms of staph produce toxins that can affect many parts of the body. Other strains are known as hemolytic, meaning that they can destroy red blood cells during an infection. In the airways, staph can cause lung abscesses and pneumonia.

Staph are increasingly resistant to penicillin and other antibiotics and require "designer" antibiotics that have been engineered to get this tenacious bacteria under control.

2. STREPTOCOCCUS PNEUMONIAE (PNEUMOCOCCUS)

This bacterium can be considered the number one bacterial enemy of the respiratory system. These gram-positive, round bacteria grow in patterns that resemble chains under a microscope. Strep pneumoniae can cause pneumonia, meningitis, sinusitis, and ear infections. Found practically everywhere in nature, they can live for years in the upper airways without causing disease. Usually they become infectious when there is a breakdown in the defenses of the host. In general they are not felt to spread from individual to individual.

Some forms of streptococcus, also called pneumococcus, are coated with a slippery capsule that allows them to evade white blood cells trying to destroy them. Doctors are particularly concerned with their increasing resistance to antibiotics.

3. STREPTOCOCCUS PYOGENES (STREP)

This is the strep that we all fear. Also called strep A or simply strep, it causes the classic strep throat. These aggressive gram-positive bacteria have specialized projections known as *pili* that allow them to stick to the mucous membranes in the throat. In addition to a very sore throat, strep pyogenes can also cause pneumonia and, indirectly, rheumatic fever and a kidney disease called glomerulonephritis.

Strep A can be found in up to 20 percent of healthy children, but its presence in adults indicates an active infection. Over ninety different types of *Streptococcus pyogenes* exist, and it is hard to develop immunity to this widespread bacteria. It is easily spread by droplets in the air, and unlike most bacteria it causes widespread tissue damage in the body.

Strep responds well to many of the widely used antibiotics, but has shown increasing resistance to penicillin and erythromycin.

4. Haemophilus influenzae (Hib)

In the 1840s, doctors thought that this bacteria caused influenza. More than one hundred years later, the flu virus was finally isolated and identified, but this bacteria retained its name. These small aerobic, gram-negative bacteria frequently live harmlessly in the upper airways.

There are two types of *Haemophilus influenzae*, a and b. The most dangerous form is Haemophilus b which is protected by a capsule that shields it from our defensive white blood cells. This is the form of Hi that causes meningitis in children. Fortunately, a vaccine is now routinely given as part of childhood immunization that prevents this deadly disease.

The nonencapsulated forms of Hi can cause sinusitis, ear infections, and bronchitis in adults with underlying chronic lung disease.

5. Klebsiella pneumoniae

There are more than eighty types of these large gram-negative rods. They commonly cause urinary tract infections, but may also cause severe pneumonia that can lead to permanent lung damage. When it does affect the respiratory tract, klebsiella can spread to other parts of the body, by a type of infection known as *bacteremia*. Klebsiella pneumonia is usually seen in people with a history of alcoholism and chronic lung disease. Because klebsiella infections can spread rapidly, doctors often use a combination of antibiotics to treat it. These organisms tend to be resistant to penicillin, but can be vanquished with newer antibiotics.

6. Pseudomonas aeruginosa

Doctors have identified over one hundred different species of these aerobic, gram-negative bacteria. Pseudomonas live in moist environments such as soil and water. They usually cause infections in people who are already hospitalized for other reasons, and these bacteria are unfortunately resistant to most antibiotics. This is the one type of pneumonia where identification of the bacteria is important in order to select the most effective combination of antibiotics.

7. CHLAMYDIA PNEUMONIAE

These organisms have unique characteristics that distinguish them from other bacteria. It is estimated that 60–80 percent of people become infected with C. pneumoniae during their lifetime, but it is rarely diagnosed. In addition to causing pneumonia, bronchitis, and sinusitis, these bacteria are believed to be an important trigger of asthmatic attacks in susceptible people. There have also been troubling studies that indicate that C. pneumoniae can increase plaque formation in the arteries, leading to increased incidence of heart attacks.

C. pneumoniae is slow to reproduce, and it can take three weeks after exposure to develop symptoms of a respiratory infection. Unlike many of the common bacterial pneumonias, such as that caused by Streptococcus pneumoniae, C. pneumoniae spreads from person to person, leading to small epidemics, and there have been some dramatic outbreaks of C. pneumoniae in Scandinavian schools and military camps.

Because of its growth patterns, this iconoclastic organism often needs three weeks of antibiotic therapy rather than the usual five-to-seven-day course.

8. LEGIONELLA PNEUMOPHILA
(LEGIONNAIRE'S BACILLUS)

First identified in 1976, after an outbreak of pneumonia affected almost two hundred people at a Legionnaire's convention in Philadelphia, Legionella bacteria love water. They have been found in pools of water in air-conditioning systems, in the hot-water systems of hospitals and hotels, in swirling whirlpools at spas, and even in the nozzles of health club showers. Legionella produces an especially severe pneumonia that can affect large areas of both lungs, and kidney failure is a frequent complication. These gram-negative rods are usually active in late summer and early autumn. Because they frequently contaminate air-conditioning systems, they can produce a small, contained epidemic.

VIRUSES—THE INVISIBLE ENEMY

Viruses are the terrorists of the microbial world. Relentless, secretive, and lethal, they are focused on a single purpose—finding new living cells to attack and destroy. Viral diseases have plagued humans for centuries, causing widespread disease that has changed the course of human history. Historians believe that smallpox contributed to the fall of the Roman Empire, and that the influenza epidemic of 1918–19 may have shortened World War I.

In the nineteenth century, scientists were making great strides in identifying the bacterial causes of disease. To isolate these organisms, they used unglazed porcelain filters to separate and concentrate disease-causing microbes. These filters had pores so tiny that no organism known at that time could pass through. In 1882, however, a Russian botanist found that the experimental fluid that had passed through his filters could still cause a destructive disease in tobacco plants. A few years later, a Dutch researcher demonstrated the same phenomenon with the organism that causes hoof-and-mouth disease in cattle.

These agents were called filterable viruses, since they passed through filters through which no bacteria could penetrate. Further investigations showed that these newly defined organisms were responsible for a wide range of diseases including smallpox, rabies, measles, mumps, herpes, polio, and chicken pox.

Knowledge about viruses and the diseases they cause came in fits and starts. Invisible in traditional microscopes and impossible to grow in culture media, viruses defied study and control. In 1925 when the newly developed electron microscope finally allowed scientists to see a virus, they were shocked. These tiny killers were minute crystalline structures, looking much more like salt than living, growing organisms. Finally in 1931, scientists were able to grow influenza virus in chicken embryos. It had been little more than a decade since the devastating influenza pandemic in the closing days of World War I, and the isolation of a live influenza virus was met with equal measures of joy and relief.

Viruses are too small to be seen with a standard laboratory microscope and need living cells in order to survive. A virus attaches to a cell, inserts genetic material, and takes over the cell. Once inside the cell nucleus, the virus begins to reproduce. When the new viral particles are formed, they burst out of the cell. The new viruses rush out of the now dead cell to find new victims in the body.

Viruses tend to favor specific types of cells. For example, the polio virus attacks the central nervous system, while herpes simplex targets skin and mucous membranes. Some of the most common viruses that cause disease in humans make their home in the nose, throat, and lungs.

Viruses are extremely difficult to control. They are tiny, primitive organisms that provide few targets for treatment. By contrast, bacteria are fully formed organisms with a wide range of activities. We have been able to develop agents such as antibiotics that can, either singly or in combination, target reproduction, metabolism, or even their attachment mechanism to the human cell. Viruses are only alive and active while they are in a cell, and drugs strong enough to kill them are usually toxic to the rest of the body. In recent years we have developed a few antiviral agents, but our best defense against viruses is a good offense with vaccination.

In the decades since the first virus was isolated, over eighty groups of viruses that cause human disease have been identified. Of these, just three major groups attack the upper and/or lower airways:

1. COLD VIRUSES

To date, more than two hundred types of cold viruses belonging to seven different groups have been identified. Some tend to affect children more than adults; others cause illness in the winter, while some types appear in the spring. Cold viruses vary in the way they are spread. For example, rhinoviruses are transmitted by direct contact, while the corona cold virus is communicated by droplets in the air.

2. INFLUENZA VIRUSES

There are three basic types of influenza viruses, designated as A, B, and C. Each lettered group has specific characteristics, but they all share one important trait, called *genetic drift*. This simply means that influenza viruses change their genetic makeup from year to year. To survive, the influenza virus needs to attack a living cell. When a virus attacks, our bodies develop antibodies against that particular virus and fight off and limit disease. The next time that virus invades, it will find antibodies already in the body to stop its reproduction. To survive, viruses change their genetic coding just enough so that the existing antibodies cannot recognize them. In some years these genetic changes can make the flu more aggressive and cause increased damage to the airways.

3. RESPIRATORY SYNCYTIAL VIRUS (RSV)

This widespread virus usually causes mild illness in children. In fact, by the age of three, most children have had a mild upper-respiratory RSV infection. However, if RSV infection travels to the lower respiratory system (the small bronchi and the lungs), it can cause severe diseases such as bronchiolitis and pneumonia. Severe RSV infection in early childhood may increase the risk of developing asthma. Studies have shown that up to 50 percent of infants hospitalized with RSV may go on to develop pneumonia.

RSV, which usually appears in late fall and winter, is spread by close contact via saliva droplets. The virus can also live for hours on such objects as doorknobs, telephones, and handrails of stairs.

MYCOPLASMA PNEUMONIAE— THE OTHER MICROORGANISM

Myclopasma are the smallest organisms that can grow outside a cell. First isolated from cattle suffering from pneumonia, scientists have now identified five distinct types and over 150 species. Mycoplasma are midway in size and characteristics between a virus and a bacterium. They can reproduce by dividing like bacteria, but they are about the size of a large virus.

Mycoplasma come in a variety of shapes. They can be round, hollow rings, branching filaments, and even dumbbell-shaped. In the respiratory system mycoplasma cause a mild but lingering pneumonia. It is believed that more than 15 percent of pneumonias are due to this little-understood organism. The good news about mycoplasma is that it responds to the newer antibiotics.

CHAPTER 3

TREATMENT—THE RIGHT CHOICE AT THE RIGHT TIME

While it's true we don't have a single silver bullet to cure colds, flu, and other respiratory infections, there are ten different treatment options that singly or in combination can prevent, treat, and shorten the duration of discomfort. Each type of treatment deals with an individual cluster of symptoms and problems. When you understand how each treatment works, you will be able to manage your respiratory infections safely, affordably, and comfortably. The challenge is knowing how and when to use them.

Antihistamines—How to Stop Sneezing and Cope with a Cold

Histamine is a natural body chemical that produces a number of changes in the body, including inflammation. Inflammation is characterized by redness (which indicates that blood is coming to the inflamed tissues), swelling (which means that fluid has leaked into the tissue), and pain (a sign that chemicals have been released into the tissues, which triggers reactions from the nerve endings).

It is well-known that histamine is a major player in allergies, where it causes mucus production, tissue swelling, and narrowing of the airways, but what is less well-known is the role of histamine in viral infections such as colds and flu. Viruses provoke the release of inflammatory compounds such as histamine that produce the unwanted, all-too-familiar sneezing, throat pain, and congestion of a cold. Antihistamines limit the action of these compounds, short-circuiting unnecessary inflammatory consequences.

There are two types of antihistamines. The older, first-generation antihistamines, such as chlorpheniramine (trade name Chlor-Trimeton), clemastine (trade name Tavist), and diphenhydramine (trade name Benadryl), have been used for more than forty years. They're extremely effective, but they can cause drowsiness. The newer, second generation of antihistamines, such as Fexofenadine (Allegra) and loratadine (Claritin), are equally effective for allergies, and because they do not cross the blood-brain barrier, they do not make you sleepy. However, they may be less effective for cold and flu symptoms.

Some people do not get sleepy from any type of antihistamine, and they can take them during the day or night. Others find that traditional antihistamines make them groggy and reserve them for the evening to relieve nighttime congestion and ensure a good night's sleep.

Antihistamines are one of the most important weapons in the cold and flu arsenal to relieve discomfort. They provide control of congestion, sneezing, and even cough. They're inexpensive, widely available, and have a low incidence of unpleasant side effects. Because they work so well, one tends to take too many, and higher doses can cause dry throat and nasal passages, which can be irritating. Do not exceed the recommended dosage on the package. Keep in mind that combination products usually contain antihistamines, and it is not wise to add additional cold-care remedies when taking combination products.

Decongestants—Breathing Easy Again

We all know the term, but do we know how decongestants work? Basically, decongestants relieve pressure and congestion not by drying up mucus, but by shrinking blood vessels in the nose so that they don't block the airways. The cold virus provokes the release of inflammatory compounds that swell the tiny vessels in the nasal passages. Given that it's already a small space, even small increases in the size of blood vessels can cause congestion and difficulty in breathing.

There are three types of decongestants. Alpha agonists such as *pseudoephedrines* (found in Sudafed and Actifed) are widely used medications. These act by contracting smooth muscle in blood vessels, shrinking the vessels and allowing you to breathe easier. They are available in pills and syrups. Because they shrink blood vessels, oral decongestants can raise blood pressure and heart rate, make you feel jittery, or cause insomnia. If you have high blood pressure or a cardiac condition, consult your doctor before taking these medications. They should be used in the morning rather than at night, so as not to interfere with sleep.

Decongestants are also effective in the form of a spray (Afrin). Applied directly to swollen tissues, they shrink them almost immediately and relieve congestion. However, overuse can cause what is known as rebound congestion. Because the sprays work so fast and so well, people tend to use them past the three-day limit recommended on the package label. As the spray wears off, the tiny blood vessels in the nose expand, leading to feelings of congestion. It is so uncomfortable that the decongestant sprays are used again. This overusage can lead to a dependency that can last for years. Sometimes the addiction is so intense that withdrawal requires the help of an ear and nose specialist. To prevent this problem, do not use decongestant sprays for more than three days in a row. If you become congested from a cold or flu, try using a decongestant spray for the first few days, then switch to the oral form for the rest of the illness.

The second type of decongestants are called *anticholinergics*. These act by blocking the body chemical called acetylcholine which both stimulates mucous glands and relaxes smooth muscles in blood vessels. While it is good to have relaxed muscles in your back and neck, relaxed smooth muscles in the blood vessels of the nose can cause congestion. By blocking the local production of acetylcholine, you can decrease mucus production and shrink swollen blood vessels. Anticholinergic decongestants are only available in a nasal spray such as Atrovent. While they do not cause rebound congestion, they have been known to cause dryness or even nosebleeds. If this happens, you can moisten the nasal mucosa with saline spray or try to reduce the number of times you use this product. Failing this, another decongestant should be tried.

The third type of decongestants are aromatic chemicals such as camphor, eucalyptus oil, mustard, tincture of benzoin, and menthol. They relieve congestion by stimulating the mucous glands in the nose to produce more fluid. This thin mucus softens and dilutes the dry, hardened mucus already causing congestion. As a result, it becomes easier for the airways to clear themselves of congestion via coughing or nose blowing. This type of decongestant is almost as old as medicine itself and is still successfully used around the world. Some of these ingredients, such as menthol, are used in sprays and lozenges. Others, such as tincture of benzoin and eucalyptus leaves, are inhaled in a vaporizer. Camphor and mustard are found in traditional chest rubs. Modern medicine debates the value of these remedies, but for many people they offer gentle relief. However, if you have allergies, asthma, emphysema, or other chronic lung disorders, it is wise to stay from any treatment that contains these irritating compounds.

Pain Relief—the Foundation of Cold and Flu Care

Headache, fever, and body aches are three characteristic symptoms of respiratory infections. These discomforts are the result of the bacterial- and viral-induced production of inflammatory compounds by the body. The microorganisms stimulate our defense mechanisms, which in turn release chemical mediators. The most prevalent of these compounds are the prostaglandins. It's not clear how effective these mediators are in fighting disease, but we do know they are responsible for unwanted symptoms such as fever and body aches. Fortunately, we have three types of anti-inflammatory agents that offer long-lasting relief from prostaglandins and other inflammatory mediators by blocking their production.

A New Respect for an Old Drug

"Take two aspirin and call me in the morning." This phrase is an old cliché, but aspirin is truly an extraordinary and effective medication. Chemically, aspirin is a salicylate, originally derived from willow bark. The therapeutic value of this natural remedy has been known for centuries by many different cultures. In eighteenth-century England, the Reverend Edmund Stone wrote to the Royal Society that the bark of the willow will cure "agues" or fever. He reasoned that because the willow grew in damp areas, it would probably possess curative therapeutic properties opposite to the dampness.

The active ingredient in aspirin is salasin. It was first isolated in 1829, when its fever-reducing properties were demonstrated. It was introduced commercially in 1899 by a chemist working for the Bayer pharmaceutical company. The name *aspirin* was derived from spirea, a plant from which salicylic acid was once prepared.

Aspirin is inexpensive and available everywhere in the world, but it is not without a few drawbacks. As an acid, it can be irritating to the lining of the stomach. This can produce a burning sensation, acidity, and reflux (the regurgitation of stomach acid into the esophagus). If you take large amounts of aspirin over several months, it can cause a peptic ulcer. Aspirin has additional toxicity. If you take more than the daily recommended dosage, you can develop gastrointestinal problems. Aspirin should be avoided by asthmatics because of the frequency of serious allergic reactions it can cause in them. It should not be used in children or young adults during a viral infection, due to increased risk of Reye's syndrome, a severe neurological syndrome that can follow a viral infection.

Acetaminophen, commonly sold under the trade name Tylenol, was introduced in 1955, originally intended for relief of pain and fever in children. It proved so safe and effective it was soon recommended for adult discomfort as well. It is characterized as a nonnarcotic antipain, antifever medication. Strictly speaking, it is not considered an anti-inflammatory agent, although it is believed to inhibit prostaglandins. Tylenol does not cause gastric upset and bleeding problems like aspirin, but can cause liver damage if taken in high doses. Tylenol can safely be taken during pregnancy, by people with aspirin sensitivity and ulcers, as well as by those on medications that thin the blood. Because of the link to liver damage, Tylenol should be avoided by those with a history of alcohol abuse or hepatitis.

Adults can safely take five hundred to a thousand milligrams of Tylenol up to four times a day. Relief of pain and fever usually lasts for three to four hours. When choosing cold-care products, keep in mind that many combination drugs contain acetaminophen, and if they're taken together with acetaminophen, it is possible to ingest excessive amounts of this drug. Reading labels will be helpful. But a number of products list acetaminophen in ways that are not easily recognizable. To avoid potential problems, if you take a combination cold product, don't take additional acetaminophen, or other combination drugs.

Ibuprofen, found in Advil and Motrin, relieves fever, headache, and body aches by inhibiting inflammatory prostaglandins. This effective, widely used drug is characterized as a nonsteroidal anti-inflammatory, or NSAID. Ibuprofen was originally introduced as a prescription drug and was later made available over the counter. Considered as effective for pain relief as aspirin and acetaminophen, it causes less bleeding problems than aspirin. Unlike with narcotic pain relievers, happily, you don't develop a dependency on it. However, peptic ulcers and kidney damage can occur with chronic use. For these reasons, doctors warn that people with peptic ulcers, a history of alcohol abuse, or those over age seventy use acetominophen to avoid complications from ibuprofen.

When colds do strike, you can take four hundred milligrams of ibuprofen up to three times a day. Keep in mind that NSAIDs decrease kidney blood flow, which can lead to fluid retention and hypertension. If you have congestive heart failure or kidney problems, your doctor may suggest avoiding ibuprofen.

As mentioned, cold and flu viruses cause the body to release different cell mediators that produce different types of inflammation. The prostaglandins are felt to be responsible for fever and pain. Fever is a natural defense against disease, but it is a double-edged sword. Fever increases *free radicals* (harmful chemicals that form as the result of tissue damage and inflammation), raises blood pressure, increases dehydration, and increases headaches and body aches. When a fever exceeds one hundred degrees Fahrenheit, its drawbacks outweigh its defense benefits. We are better able to fight disease if we don't also have to deal with inflammation and fever, and it is in our best interest to take acetaminophen, aspirin, or ibuprofen to reduce fever.

Anti-inflammatory agents such as aspirin or acetaminophen are the foundation of care for respiratory infections. While they don't relieve congestion, they target aches, fever, and that general feeling of exhaustion that accompanies respiratory infections. I have found that my patients are reluctant to take them if they don't have a headache or have little fever. Once they realize that these drugs are not just for headaches, they are better able to care for any type of respiratory infection.

Quelling the Cough

The cough that accompanies most respiratory infection is annoying, exhausting, and even painful. The presence of irritants in the airways, such as mucus or inflammatory agents, triggers the cough reflex. As unwanted as it is, the cough is actually the body's mechanism to keep the airways clear and open. Rather than simply suppressing the cough, the key to cough control is to deal with the underlying causes.

When the cough results from excess mucus production (as during a cold), antihistamines and/or decongestants will remove the underlying cause of the cough. When the cough is part of pneumonia or bronchitis, antibiotics can kill the underlying bacterial infection, and the cough will end. To relieve discomfort as we treat the root of the cough, I may prescribe a cough medicine to help my patients rest.

There are four kinds of cough medicines. Cough suppressants, also known as *antitussives,* inhibit the activity in the brain that controls the cough reflex. Prescription cough suppressants contain codeine and related medications, while those that are available over the counter are formulated with dextromethorphan.

In some infections, the mucus becomes so hard and dry that it cannot be brought up by coughing. This consolidation of mucus in the chest and airways is an open invitation for bacterial infection to develop. Expectorant cough formulations thin and loosen mucus secretions, allowing them to be brought up by coughing or blowing your nose. Available without prescription, the active ingredient in many expectorants is guaifenesin.

Anesthetic cough sprays and lozenges that contain such ingredients as benzocaine or phenol act by temporarily numbing the irritated nerves in the throat that are triggering the cough reflex. The relief is almost immediate and allows you to get some much needed rest. Even a simple sugar-based cough drop offers a degree of relief. As a group they are called demulcents, and they act by coating the irritated lining of the throat with a gel-like substance. Honey, licorice, glycerin, and even corn syrup are demulcents that can soothe a cough-irritated throat. You will find that modern cough drops often are a combination of different ingredients. For example, both Listerine cough control and Vicks Formula 44 cough discs contain benzocaine (which dulls the cough nerves in the throat) and dextromethorphan (which quells the cough reflex in the brain). This provides instant as well as long-lasting relief.

Because coughing is actually a healthy reflex, I don't want you to suppress this symptom without dealing with the underlying cause. But if you're treating the cause of the cough, then the right type of cough-care product will help you feel more comfortable. You will be able to get some rest and will recover more rapidly. Cough medicines are often combined with antihistamines, decongestants, and analgesics, such as aspirin and Tylenol. These products may be less expensive than the same ingredients bought separately, and can be more convenient at work and school. Just don't mix and match combination products or take additional single ingredients, to avoid overdosing from cold-care products.

A cough that lingers for several weeks after a respiratory infection may indicate the development of an asthmalike syndrome. The original infection has sufficiently damaged the airways so they are inflamed and irritable. Substances in the environment that once did not cause a problem (such as cigarette smoke, perfume, pets, or even cold air) now trigger contraction of the airways, causing you to cough. The most effective way to manage this cough is to use the same type of bronchodilator that is used successfully for true asthma.

Two types of bronchodilators work well for this type of cough. Each acts on separate factors in the cells that cause airways to narrow. *Beta agonists* such as albuterol (Ventolin HFA) relax muscles in the airways. They work almost immediately and the relief lasts for hours. There are some side effects, including increased heart rate, palpitations, and insomnia. Patients with cardiovascular conditions should ask their physician about any limitation to the use of these agents. For a postcold or postflu cough, the spray may be used up to four times a day for up to six weeks.

The second type of bronchodilators are *anticholinergics,* which block the action of acetylcholine. This natural body chemical causes smooth muscles to contract. When used as an oral inhaler, anticholinergics (such as Atrovent) prevent irritable airways from narrowing, thus short-circuiting the cough reflex. These medications can cause side effects such as dry mouth.

The Truth About Antibiotics

At one time, the arrival of a cold or flu was a trigger for an automatic prescription for antibiotics. But antibiotics work for bacterial infections, not viral infections. The Centers for Disease Control and Prevention (CDC), the American Medical Association, the American Thoracic Society, and the World Health Organization have strongly encouraged doctors and patients to limit the use of antibiotics in respiratory infections, because the majority of such infections are caused by viruses. That being said, occasionally an upper and lower respiratory infection that begins as a viral infection can become superinfected with bacteria (this represents a secondary infection of damaged tissue). This is particularly true when the infection causes obstruction of draining passages, such as in the canals that drain the middle ear, or the tracts that allow the sinuses in the head to drain out during a cold. If these become obstructed, the mucus can build up and become infected with bacteria.

For generally healthy patients, I will prescribe antibiotics for respiratory infections that last longer than a week to ten days, if pain develops in the sinus area, when a fever doesn't go away and actually increases, or if there is presence of discolored or blood-tinged mucus. When there are underlying health conditions, or in small children under the age of two, the threshold for using antibiotics is significantly lower. These are situations you need to discuss with your own doctor.

There are now four excellent categories of antibiotics for the treatment of respiratory infections. The choice depends on the type of infection, whether it's in the upper respiratory tract (the throat and the nose), or if it involves the lower respiratory tract, i.e., the lungs. In addition, the choice of antibiotics depends on which bacteria may be causing the infection, your other health considerations, and the cost of the drug.

The first group, which is among the oldest of antibiotics, is called the *beta lactams*. The earliest form of these compounds were the penicillins, still widely used today. Penicillin is what is called a narrow-spectrum antibiotic. That is, it is effective against a relatively small number of organisms, particularly those that are gram-positive, such as the ones that cause strep throat or pneumococcal pneumonia. But over the years, the ability of beta lactams to fight infections has been extended to cover many other bacteria. It is also true that bacteria have learned how to outsmart beta lactams, a situation we call bacterial resistance. As a result, researchers have now modified the original molecules and attached additional compounds to the antibiotics, making them as effective as they were in the past. These additional compounds are not antibiotics in and of themselves, but help penicillin and other beta lactams to maintain their effectiveness in the face of ever-smarter bacteria.

One example of these enhanced beta lactams is Augmentin, which combines amoxicillin, a broad-spectrum penicillin, with clavulanic acid, a compound that prevents bacteria from destroying the penicillin drug. These drugs are extremely effective and are commonly prescribed in the treatment of bacterial infections of the upper respiratory tract. Augmentin, like other penicillins and beta lactams, is bactericidal, which means that it actually kills the bacteria. These drugs can be administered by injection or by mouth, but for a simple respiratory infection, I will prescribe them in pills or liquid.

In general, penicillins are well tolerated. However, a significant proportion of healthy people are allergic to penicillin, and it can actually lead to a life-threatening reaction. Some of the beta lactams, especially those that are broad-spectrum, can create some gastrointestinal problems, such as nausea and diarrhea, but these are generally mild side effects that don't cause you to stop taking the antibiotic.

The second group of antibiotics, which are actually closely related to penicillins, are the *cephalosporins*. The original compound is similar to penicillin. Examples of cephalosporin are Ceftin, Ceclor, and Rocephin. Each generation of cephalosporins was developed to meet certain needs. By and large, the more recent generations of cephalosporins are used for serious, often life-threatening illnesses and would not be used to treat an upper respiratory infection such as a sinus infection. However, these agents are effective in treating all kinds of bacteria that are found in the lower respiratory tract. Some are administered by injection or intravenously for hospitalized patients, while others can be given by mouth.

The cephalosporins have the advantage over penicillin in that they cause fewer allergic reactions. However, if someone is already sensitive to penicillin, then it is probably not a good idea for him or her to take cephalosporins, because of potential cross-reactivity for a serious anaphylactic reaction.

The third class of antibiotics used for the treatment of respiratory infections are the *macrolides*. The parent compound that spawned this whole family of macrolides was erythromycin. More recent versions of macrolides include Biaxin and Zithromax. These compounds are unrelated to penicillin, so that in general there is no allergic cross-reactivity. They are well tolerated, although mild GI side effects have been reported. They can be given intravenously and intramuscularly, but generally we can simply give them orally. The more recent compounds such as Biaxin XL and Zithromax have the advantage that they can be taken just once a day.

Unlike the beta lactam antibiotics, which kill the bacteria by preventing them from forming cell walls, the macrolides stop the bacteria from making proteins, slowing them down, so the body's natural defenses can bring them under control. Therefore in general, the macrolides are considered bacteriostatic, rather than bactericidal. Macrolides are versatile and are frequently used in the treatment of bacterial infections of the respiratory tract such as bronchitis.

The fourth class of antibiotics that are used for respiratory infections are the *quinolones*. These agents were originally used to treat urinary tract infections, but they have undergone a series of modifications that have led to multiple generations of these drugs, and the more recent ones are extremely effective in the treatment of bacteria that cause respiratory infections. These agents can be given by mouth and by injection. Common examples are Levaquin, Tequin, and Avelox. They are prescribed for strep throat (when there is a penicillin allergy), bronchitis, pneumonia, and sinusitis.

Vaccines—the "Jab" That Can Save Your Life

Although a vaccine for the cold has eluded scientists, there are safe and effective immunizations for both influenza and pneumonia.

Each time you're exposed to a specific virus, the body develops antibodies to fight the infection. When you recover, your body retains the ability to quickly manufacture these antibodies, providing immunity against another infection from the same virus. But the virus that causes influenza undergoes genetic change every year, so that the existing antibodies don't always recognize the new genetic makeup of the current flu strain. When the changes are small, they are called antigenic drifts, and the flu outbreak that year will be mild.

When the genetic changes are big, it is called an antigenic shift. When this happens, as it did in 1968 with the Hong Kong flu, the disease is worldwide and severe. Each year scientists at the World Health Organization and the Centers for Disease Control and Prevention try to anticipate the next new strain of influenza. Each annual vaccine contains antibodies for three of the new most common strains that the doctors can identify early.

In 2004, the flu vaccine contained the newly identified Fujian strain, which produces a more severe form than has occurred in recent years. In 2005, doctors are exploring the possibility of including the antigens for avian or bird flu, an especially virulent form of the flu virus. It takes twelve months of concentrated effort to identify new strains, grow them in live egg cultures, and process them for use. The vaccine is shipped to doctors in early October, and recommendations are for vaccination to start in late October and November.

The immunity lasts four to five months and weakens over time. Because the elderly are among the most likely to develop life-threatening complications, some doctors recommend a second vaccination booster in December for this vulnerable population until the flu season ends, in the last weeks of February.

There are currently two forms of flu vaccines: the trivalent (meaning "three strains") inactivated influenza virus that is indicated for people of any age and given by injection; and the trivalent live, attenuated influenza, known as LAIV, that is given by a nasal spray and is indicated for healthy people ages six to forty-nine.

WHO SHOULD GET THE FLU VACCINE?

- People aged fifty or older
- People aged six to twenty-three months
- Women who will be pregnant during the influenza season
- People aged six months to forty-nine years with any of the following conditions
  - chronic pulmonary disorder (e.g., asthma or COPD)
  - chronic heart disease
  - chronic disease of the blood (e.g., sickle-cell anemia)
  - chronic kidney disease
  - HIV
  - diabetes
  - child or teenager receiving long-term aspirin therapy
  - resides in a nursing home
  - likely to transmit influenza to persons at risk
  - household members of high-risk people

The latest guidelines for flu vaccinations were issued in 2004, and they significantly increased the CDC recommendations for who should get the vaccine.

Unfortunately, in 2004, half of the 90–100 million units of vaccine that were developed had bacterial contamination and could not be used. There was initially public panic, and long lines of frightened people waited for the few available shots. After years of begging my patients to come in for a flu shot, I was suddenly the most popular guy in my neighborhood. All of my patients, friends, neighbors, and even my dry cleaner, were asking me for the flu shot. Eventually, most of the high-risk individuals received influenza protection, and I am hoping that the increased awareness will make it easier for me to convince patients, friends, and family to come in for their shots.

The flu vaccine provides safe and effective protection. It can cause mild pain and redness around the injection site that goes away within twenty-four hours. You cannot get the flu from the flu shot, but mild, short-lived, flu-like symptoms from the body's response to the virus can develop. There is still significant public resistance to the shot. Only 65 percent of people over age sixty-five get vaccinated against the flu. Among young adults, only 12 percent of those who are at risk for complications are protected with an annual flu vaccine.

Behind the Vaccination Crisis: A Decade in Coming

In September 2004, it was discovered that one-half of the 90–100 million required doses of the flu vaccine were contaminated with bacteria. Among health practitioners, the extreme shortage of vaccine for Americans was met with dismay but not surprise. For more than a decade, virologists and public health experts had warned that the vaccine production system was seriously flawed—a potentially deadly mixture of old technology, low prices, and politics.

Vaccine production hasn't changed much since the nineteenth century when Aventis began producing vaccine commercially in Pennsylvania, a state chosen because it was the nation's leading egg producer.

Each year millions of fertilized eggs are inoculated with one of the three selected viral strains. The eggs are incubated for several days, becoming little flu factories as the virus replicates rapidly. The virus-rich egg whites are extracted, concentrated, and inactivated (or killed) by detergents. Then the three strains are blended into a single vaccine. Once it is tested and approved by the FDA, it is distributed to physicians, hospitals, and other health care facilities.

The influenza vaccine contains immunogens, inactive components of the flu virus. Immune cells in the body react to the flulike forms and start producing antibodies. These antibodies stick to the spikes that the virus uses to enter a cell, preventing it from attacking and destroying the cell.

Each egg produces one to two doses of the vaccine, and it takes six to eight months to produce enough vaccine to meet our needs. Unforeseen events can happen at each of the dozens of steps of the way. For example, there is always a bit of anxiety that the millions of eggs needed to produce the vaccine will be available.

Despite the obvious drawbacks of this old technology, high costs, low profits, and growing risk of lawsuits provide little incentive to change. Since the 1992 Childhood Immunization Act, the government buys 55 percent of the vaccine stock at greatly reduced prices that barely covers the cost of manufacture. The vaccine manufacturers don't fare much better in the private sector. Each year they produce tens of millions of doses that are unused and must be discarded. For example, from 2000 to 2003, Wyeth pharmaceuticals threw out 35 million doses of unused influenza vaccine at a loss of $50 million. Facing additional millions in costs to upgrade their factories to meet FDA standards, Wyeth decided to focus on vaccines for meningitis and pneumonia that do not need to be remade each year.

It is sobering to realize that the total annual global revenues for all vaccines is $6 billion, while worldwide drug revenues are $340 billion. Put another way, world revenue for all vaccines is 60 percent of the U.S. sales of a single cholesterol-lowering drug called Lipitor.

Damage suits against manufacturers have also plagued vaccine production. When the swine flu broke out at Fort Dix in 1976, Congress assumed liability for the nationwide vaccine program. More than four thousand lawsuits were filed against the manufacturers, seven hundred were successful, and the liability came to $100 million. To protect manufacturers and the public, Congress passed the National Vaccine Injury Compensation Program in 1986. The aim was to create a means to compensate legitimate injuries. Unlike workman's compensation, where decisions are binding, the program is not mandatory. Any party can sue if they disagree with the decisions of the board that reviews the medical circumstances of a case.

Virtually all the lawsuits against vaccine manufacturers involving thimerosal, a preservative used since the 1930s, have bypassed the board. In the 1980s some doctors and concerned parents suggested that thimerosal in vaccines was the cause of the significant rise in childhood autism. Currently, three hundred ongoing lawsuits are asking for more money than the entire annual worldwide sales of all vaccines. Moreover, the Injury Compensation Program only covers childhood vaccines, not adult vaccines such as those used against influenza.

Congress has repeatedly refused to pass legislation that would indemnify or at least limit liability for vaccine manufacturers. Thirty years ago there were twenty-five major vaccine manufacturers. Today there are just five, and only two that produce influenza vaccines in the United States. Given the economic and legal climate, it is not surprising that new influenza vaccine production developments have been slow in coming in the United States.

In Europe, both older established companies and new bioengineering start-ups are working to change their egg-based vaccine production to cell culture techniques. These have already been used to successfully produce smallpox vaccine. While a single egg can supply only one to two doses of flu vaccine, cell cultures can provide uncountable amounts of virus. Even more encouraging, it takes less time to grow cell culture virus, and vaccine can be produced to meet yearly needs. It will take both time and money to develop approved cell culture flu vaccine. It is estimated to cost upward of $250 million and to take three to four years before approval by the FDA.

And it is already underway. Baxter International is planning to use cell technology to produce a flu vaccine in the Czech Republic, using the same successful techniques that have been developed for smallpox vaccine production. Baxter plans to launch the vaccine in 2006 in Europe and seek approval in the United States at the same time. Chiron is already entering the Phase III studies of a cell culture vaccine and hopes to market it in Europe in 2007.

The 2004 flu vaccine shortage and the specter of an avian flu pandemic has focused much needed attention on the systemwide problems in current influenza vaccine production and distribution. These very real dangers may be the necessary motivation to bring the current horse-and-buggy-era vaccine production into the wireless age.

Pneumonia Vaccine–the "Other" Vaccine

During the flu shot shortage of 2004, I was finally able to convince many of my patients and friends to get the other important vaccination, the shot to provide protection against bacterial pneumonia. Currently the most serious respiratory infection, pneumonia combined with flu is currently the sixth leading cause of death in the United States. The majority of bacterial pneumonias are caused by different forms of streptococcus bacteria. The pneumonia vaccine contains twenty-three different strains of disease-causing streptococcus. It is one of the most important medical advances in the last twenty years, and one of the most underutilized. Current guidelines recommend that people with underlying health problems, as well as all those over age sixty-five, get the shot. The single injection usually conveys a lifetime immunity. If the shot is given to younger high-risk people, a second shot a decade later will maintain a high level of immunity for life.

The pneumonia vaccine is well tolerated, with no accompanying discomfort. It is inexpensive and covered in full by virtually every health care provider. But despite these advantages, fewer than 50 percent of people over age sixty-five have received the vaccination. Even more troubling, only 12 percent of

> ## WHO SHOULD GET PNEUMOCOCCAL VACCINE
>
>
> - People of any age with chronic lung disease (e.g., asthma, COPD), heart disease, kidney disorders, sickle-cell anemia, or diabetes
> - People recovering from severe illness
> - People living in nursing homes or in other chronic-care facilities
> - People aged sixty-five or older

adults aged eighteen to forty-nine who are at higher risk for pneumonia have received this potentially lifesaving shot. If you remember only one piece of advice from this book, if you fall in the category of people who should have the pneumonia vaccine, please follow the recommendation to get this important shot.

Flu Busters—Drugs That Attack the Flu Virus

Influenza is one of the few viral infections for which there is a specific medication. There are two categories. Amantadine and rimantadine are used to prevent and treat flu caused by influenza A viruses, but not influenza B viruses. They can be used preventively in people who did not get the flu shot, or in addition to increase immunity to people who are especially vulnerable to the flu. These could include people who are over age seventy, who have severe underlying health problems, such as those undergoing chemotherapy, who are on oxygen, or who have disabilities. These medications need to be taken daily for the duration of the flu outbreak, usually six to eight weeks. If the flu does develop, both of these drugs can be used for three to seven days to reduce symptoms and hasten recovery. Studies have shown that they provide a 50 percent reduction in the signs and symptoms of the flu. Amantadine can cause insomnia, anxiety, and jitteriness, but rimantadine is as effective and seems to cause fewer side effects.

Oseltamivir (trade name Tamiflu) and zanamivir (trade name Relenza) are neuraminidase inhibitors that actually inhibit viral replication of both influenza A and B viruses. They can be used to prevent as well as treat both types of influenza. Oseltamivir may cause gastrointestinal problems in a small number of patients. Because zanamivir can cause shortness of breath and a decline in lung function, it should not be used in people with asthma and COPD. Like amantadine and rimantadine, these two antivirals can be used either to prevent infection or to treat an infection once it has started.

All categories of antiviral drugs must be taken within the first forty-eight hours of infection. If you don't get the flu shot, ask your doctor if it may be a good idea to have a supply of Tamiflu, which affects both strains A and B, in your house, to help deal with symptoms if the flu does strike.

Nutritional Therapy—Eating to Heal

"Feed a cold, starve a fever"? It's not that simple. During an infection, the body needs both nutrients and fluids to maintain strength and immunity. Doctors recommend eight glasses of water a day during health, and in illness, fluid needs increase. Fluid is needed to replace water lost from fever, as well as to thin mucus. This fluid intake can be in the form of water, tea, both hot and cold, juice, and even diet soda.

Both hot and cold water are beneficial. Cold water is more easily absorbed by the body, and hot liquids dissolve mucus. Chicken vegetable soup, the "Jewish penicillin," is a time-honored cold treatment. It provides easily digested protein, while its hot liquid thins mucus in the airways. More recently, studies have shown that chicken soup actually has an anti-inflammatory effect. Most of the common symptoms of a respiratory infection are due to the inflammatory processes provoked by the virus. Colds are associated with the production of white blood cells called neutrophils, and these cells are associated with an increase in mucus production. My colleague and friend Dr. Steven Renard at the University of Nebraska found that chicken soup actually inhibited the production of neutrophils and could possibly cause a decrease in mucus production.

Hot chicken soup is not the only hot liquid for respiratory infections. Different types of hot tea can be good sources of moisture and antioxidants (substances that protect against oxidants such as free radicals), while the heat can thin mucus. In addition, tea contains theobromine, which is a natural bronchodilator that can relieve cough. Honey and lemon added to a cup of tea have additional benefits. Both have mild antibacterial activity, and they are immediately soothing to the throat. The lemon may actually dissolve some of the virus and bacteria-laden mucus, while the honey provides a soothing coating for raw, inflamed tissues. I recommend three to four cups of hot tea throughout the day when you come down with a respiratory infection. I urge coffee drinkers to switch to tea for the duration of their symptoms. The high acid and caffeine levels of even the most delicious coffee may cause heartburn or anxiety, especially when combined with aspirin and decongestants.

Cold foods, such as sherbet, ice cream, and pudding, are helpful if you have a sore throat, or if your stomach is upset. Cold foods can be easier to digest comfortably if there are gastrointestinal problems accompanying a cold or flu. The cold temperature can also temporarily numb a sore throat, while providing easily absorbed fluid. Other easily digested foods that can be on your menu include toast, both hot and cold cereals, and scrambled eggs.

On the other end of the scale, some doctors, like my friend Dr. Irwin Ziment of UCLA, recommend spicy foods for reducing mucus congestion. Dr. Ziment believes that foods like hot-

and-sour soup, mulligatawny, or a Virgin Mary with horse-radish can provide sinus-clearing relief.

Hydrotherapy—the Water Cure

My mother decided that the best way to celebrate her seventy-fifth birthday was a trip to China. Never one to stand on the sidelines, she climbed the stones of the Great Wall of China—and fell off. When she came home, her knee was still swollen. After X-rays showed no real damage, her physician suggested rest and cold packs to the area. A few months later, when her back became sore and tight, the same physician recommended damp heat packs. In the spring, when seasonal allergies struck, her allergist recommended hot showers to clear her sinuses. She called me. "Water again," she complained. "What is it with you doctors? First it's cold water, then it's hot water. Can't you think of any other treatment but water?"

Water seems to be unimpressive, but in different forms and at different temperatures, water or hydrotherapy can provide significant help for a wide range of health problems. From steam to ice, water can be invaluable for respiratory infections. Steam, either via a sauna, a portable sauna, or just in a hot shower, melts dry, hardened mucus and will reduce congestion. A lukewarm shower can reduce fever naturally. On the other end of the scale, ice packs can temporarily relieve some of the pain and swelling of sinus infections, and ice cream can relieve sore throats. Cold water is more easily absorbed by the body than room-temperature liquids.

Saline rinses of the throat and nose can be helpful for relieving upper respiratory infections. Saline nasal rinses dissolve bacteria-laden mucus and have actually become an important part of the treatment of chronic sinusitis. You can take advantage of the benefits of saline rinses in three ways. You can make your own solution with one-quarter teaspoon salt to one cup warm water and, using a nasal bulb available at a pharmacy, simply spray the water up the nose, let it run out, then blow your nose gently. Commercially available sprays save you the trouble of mixing and filling a syringe. For chronic sinusitis, an electronic nebulizer sprays saline and other medication into the nose. This is the most expensive option, but it is covered by most health insurance plans for chronic sinusitis. All of these techniques should be done over a sink.

Gargling with saline washes away layers of virus and bacteria-laden mucus in the throat, relieving congestion and inflammation. It certainly doesn't cure the cold or sore throat, but it provides instant and welcome relief, and it may lessen the duration of the infection as you lower the amount of bacteria or viruses in the airways. Simply add one-half teaspoon table salt to warm water, gargle for ten seconds, spit, and rinse with cool water. It sounds so simplistic, but once you try it, you will become a believer.

Portable room humidifiers can be part of hydrotherapy. Cold, dry air irritates the airways, increasing risk for infection. Portable room humidifiers can relieve nasal congestion if a cold does develop. They are useful for adults and considered essential for children by many pediatricians. When using a room humidifier, it is important to follow a few simple safety tips:

- Do not let water sit unused in the tank.
- Rinse the tank out daily and wipe dry before filling with fresh water.
- If you use a cleaning solution in the tank, rinse out with several changes of fresh water before running the machine again.
- Use a hygrometer (available in hardware stores) to measure humidity in your home. While humidity below 35 percent can lead to dry, irritated airways, overhumidifying the air brings other problems. Indoor humidity over 50 percent can lead to growth of molds, bacteria, and

dust mites, all of which can increase breathing problems.
· Do not let the area around the humidifier become damp.
  Check for moisture in the rugs, carpets, and furniture
  near the machine.
· Finally, always unplug the humidifier when cleaning and
  filling it with fresh water.

Supplementing Cold and Flu Care

More interest and confusion surrounds the value of supplements for colds, flus, and other respiratory infections than all
the other treatments combined. Vitamins, herbs, flowers, min-
erals, and amino acids have all been offered as natural-care options. When choosing such remedies, it is important to
recognize both their benefits and drawbacks. It is equally essential to ask for and expect solid studies demonstrating their
disease-fighting capabilities. Out of a smorgasbord of natural
options, five have been extensively studied.

ECHINACEA: Also called snakeroot or cornflower, echinacea
belongs to the daisy family. For centuries the Plains Indians
used echinacea in poultices and teas as their primary medicine.
Three different species are approved for medical use in Europe,
and more than 1 million prescriptions for echinacea are written
yearly in Germany alone. But can 1 million Germans be wrong?

There are conflicting studies on the value or the effects of
echinacea on the prevention and treatment of colds. Supporters
believe echinacea in some way stimulates the body's own defense system. Some doctors suggest that the herb increases
phagocytosis, the gobbling up of invading bacteria and viruses
by the white blood cells. Others theorize echinacea may spur
the production of interferon, the body's own natural viral
killer. But these are just theories, and the most recent and comprehensive trials have failed to demonstrate a benefit from echinacea.

Those who believe in echinacea feel that part of the confusion over its value comes from a lack of uniformity in the actual products. Some echinacea remedies are made from the stem, others from the roots, or even a mixture of all the parts of the plant. In any event, echinacea has few side effects, except in people with allergies to pollen. It's hard to recommend something where there's so little standardization, but because it has few side effects, I don't discourage my patients from taking it as long as they use other treatments such as anti-inflammatories, antihistamines, and decongestants that have been demonstrated to improve symptoms and prevent complications.

ZINC: Zinc is a micronutrient that is needed in the healthy diet. The recommended daily allowance is twelve to fifteen milligrams per day, an amount easily met by a single serving of red meat, poultry, milk, or eggs. In these days of high-protein, low-carb diets, it's hard to imagine widespread zinc deficiency to be a national problem. However, a number of clinical trials have indicated that zinc can prevent and reduce the duration of a cold. In a study done in England and published in the *Annals of Internal Medicine,* volunteers treated with zinc lozenges had colds that lasted four days. Those volunteers who did not take the zinc lozenges continued to sniffle and sneeze for eight days. Zinc nasal spray provided similar benefits. A study done at the prestigious Cleveland Clinic found that people who used zinc spray cut the duration of their cold from six to three days.

We know that the rhinovirus uses a compound called intracellular adhesion molecule (ICAM-1) to attach and enter our cells. It is thought that zinc interferes with the production of ICAM-1 and thus prevents viral replication. Other studies suggest that zinc may strengthen cell membranes against viral invasion. Although other clinical studies did not show benefits, there is enough information about the activity of zinc on the molecular level to make doctors feel comfortable recommending zinc in cold management.

Two different forms of zinc compounds are used for colds: zinc gluconate, which can have a distinctly unpleasant taste, and zinc acetate, which is tasteless. There are dueling studies about which form works best, but there is no definitive answer. Most products that are available use zinc gluconate. Zinc cold-care products are available in four forms:

NASAL SPRAY: Misting the zinc into the nose directly treats the cells that are the first to be attacked by the cold virus. If replication can be prevented, the cold may not develop further. Zinc sprays are particularly effective when used at the very first sign of the cold—that little tickle at the back of your throat or the first few sneezes. Zinc sprays can be used every two hours to slow a cold's progression.

NASAL SWABS: They look like plain cotton swabs but are saturated with a single dose of zinc gluconate They apply virus-fighting zinc directly on the nasal tissues where the cold viruses start to grow. As you sniff, the zinc is carried slightly higher up into the nasal cavities. The recommended use is every two to four hours.

ZINC LOZENGES: These candylike tablets or balls release zinc slowly into the viral-affected and irritated throat. This is where the virus is rapidly replicating in the early stages of a cold, causing pain and inflammation and sending new particles down to the lower airways. It is hoped that using zinc lozenges every few hours will slow replication, and some clinical trials indicate that both the degree of cold symptoms and duration of the cold are shortened by their use. Look for lozenges that contain ten to twenty-five milligrams of zinc per lozenge.

ZINC PILLS: This form of zinc is not recommended. They can cause nausea, toxicity, and don't bring the zinc directly to the respiratory system where the viruses are growing. Stay away from this form of zinc.

Zinc cold therapy has been known to cause nausea, especially if you exceed recommended doses. To avoid problems, do not take zinc on an empty stomach or with citrus juice.

Vitamin C: Also known as ascorbic acid, this is a water-soluble vitamin. A diet low in vitamin C has been linked to lower immunity and bleeding gums, a condition known as scurvy. Vitamin C deficiencies have been identified for centuries. Scurvy was described in ancient Egyptian, Greek, and Roman writings. It was a leading cause of illness during the American Civil War, the exploration of the north pole, and in sailors on long sea voyages. The eighteenth-century seaman Captain James Cook was one of the first people to recognize and demonstrate that scurvy could be prevented by a diet rich in vegetables.

In the 1970s, Dr. Linus Pauling, a two-time winner of the Nobel Prize, wrote a highly controversial book claiming that large doses of vitamin C could prevent and treat a cold. The publication of the book launched literally hundreds of studies. Now, more than thirty years later, there is still no clear-cut evidence that vitamin C is the long-sought cure for a cold. The most recent and carefully controlled studies indicate that vitamin C may shorten duration of a cold somewhat and may make the symptoms less severe, but no study has demonstrated that taking vitamin C works prophylactically.

Statistically, the differences among people who take vitamin C and those who don't are small, but for an individual the impact may be much more noticeable. Vitamin C advocates suggest that with over two hundred cold viruses, some cold viruses may be affected by vitamin C while others are not, and this kind of differentiation has contributed to the conflicting study results.

Reaching for a glass of orange juice at the first sign of a

cold has become an automatic reflex, and although we don't know vitamin C's role in the treatment or management of a cold, it's not inappropriate. A viral infection like a cold can create oxidative stress in the body, leading to the development of unwanted free radicals. As a powerful antioxidant, vitamin C can reduce any radicals already formed and block new ones from developing.

A glass of nutrient-rich orange juice also provides vitamins, fluids, and easily digested calories and can therefore be an excellent choice during a cold. By contrast, the ultrahigh levels of vitamin C supplements suggested for cold prevention can be troubling to most physicians. Vitamin C advocates suggest daily doses of one thousand to three thousand milligrams, fifteen to fifty times the recommended daily allowance of sixty milligrams a day.

This level of vitamin C can be hard on your stomach. Remember, vitamin C is ascorbic acid, and this level of acidity can cause a burning feeling and indigestion. While we can't always demonstrate its value against colds, we do know that this level of vitamin C can definitely cause diarrhea. In addition, high levels of vitamins have been shown to cause antioxidant stress, just the opposite of what we want. Some researchers have suggested that the failure of the clinical trials with vitamin A and vitamin E to reduce heart disease and cancer may be linked to their unwanted increase in free radicals.

When it comes to colds, I've also found that some of my patients place too much faith in vitamin C and don't take advantage of the well-established benefits of the anti-inflammatory medications, antihistamines, and decongestants that we know work so well. I would like to see you get your vitamin C naturally in a big glass of OJ. If you want to take vitamin C, do not exceed 250 to 500 milligrams a day during a cold.

ELDERBERRY: This dark red berry has been used for centuries for a therapeutic tea. Romans brewed cups of ripe-elderberry tea as a flu remedy. While some studies have shown that elder-berry tea can reduce symptoms of a flu, keep in mind that the leaves, stems, bark, roots, and unripe berries of the plant are poisonous. Since there is no way of knowing what is in a commercially available preparation, my advice would be to avoid this alternative therapy.

GOLDENSEAL: This old-time remedy grows wild on the forest floor in North America. It was used by Cherokee Indians as an eyewash and wound cleaner. Herbalists believe that it increases immunity and recommend goldenseal tea for sore throats and diarrhea. However, few research studies back their claims. Goldenseal has been shown to increase blood pressure, as well as cause nausea and even convulsions. It may also interfere with blood clotting and should carefully be avoided by pregnant women.

Putting It All Together

Each time I go to a pharmacy, I know that if I go over to the cold and flu aisle, I will find someone scanning the shelves anxiously. Sneezing and coughing, the person picks up one box, reads the label, puts it back, then picks up another. This chapter provides the information you need to never be that person again. It explains how each item works and why it is prescribed or recommended. In addition, to help you spend less time in the cold and flu aisle, in the upcoming chapters I include a detailed treatment plan for each respiratory infection. The charts explain what components you need and the best way to take them.

The Good Doctor's Cold and Flu Survival Kit

When a cold or flu develops, it is important to have a complete stock of the supplies that you will need to deal with the symptoms. When your head feels like a block of wood and you are sneezing convulsively, the last thing you want to do is go outside and track down chicken soups and decongestants. I recommend filling a box with all the items you and your family might need when germs arrive at your home. In this box you should have:

- Acetaminophen, ibuprofen, or aspirin
- A selection of cough drops—plain, menthol, and fortified with cough surpressant
- Antihistamines
- Decongestants—both pills and spray
- Combination cold and flu care formulation to take in purse or briefcase
- Cough syrup
- Zinc lozenges and nasal spray
- Saline nasal rinse
- Packet of salt and nasal spray container
- Digital thermometer
- Vitamin C—250 mg tablets
- Waterless hand sanitizer
- Sanitizing household spray
- Tissues
- Chicken soup
- Tea bags
- Diet ginger ale and cola

If you have children under age twelve in the home, you should also have on hand:

- Children's acetaminophen or ibuprofen (no aspirin)
- Children's cough syrup
- Children's antihistamine
- Children's decongestant
- Fluid replacement solutions

- Sugar-free lollipops
- Pediatric nasal bulb
- Room humidifier
- Rectal thermometer
- Small notebook to record medications

CHAPTER 4

COLDS 101

t had been a hard year for Mrs. Salazar. A lingering cough had brought her to my office, and an X-ray showed a mass in the right lung. Surgery and chemotherapy had been successful, but the rigorous therapy had taken its toll on the fifty-seven-year-old woman. Six months later, she sat in my office, strong and healthy. She was accompanied by one of her three striking daughters, who was thrilled at her mother's recovery but was herself miserable with a chest cold. "Can't you help her?" Mrs. Salazar asked me, putting her hand on her daughter's shoulder. "You cured my cancer. Why can't you cure an ordinary cold?"

That's a good question. According to the National Health Survey, Americans get 1 billion colds a year. By definition, a cold is a mild, self-limiting disease. Adults get two to four a year, while children sneeze and cough with six to eight episodes of cold yearly. While not usually medically serious problems, colds have a huge impact on our economy, our educational system, and even our lifestyle. Colds are annually responsible for 26 million lost workdays and $3.5 billion in lost productivity. In fact, up to 40 percent of all absences from work are due to colds. Colds also affect the learning potential of our children and are responsible for 23 million absences. Colds are a problem for the military, with estimates that up to 20 percent of recruits become ill with a cold during basic training, and upper respiratory infections are a big problem in military operations. Colds also arrive at inconvenient times. My patients have included sneezing brides, coughing radio announcers, even an opera singer who had lost her voice before the start of the season.

Colds are such a part of our lives that a complete vocabulary exists to describe each stage of a cold. In the beginning, we are "catching" or "coming down with a cold." As symptoms progress, we are now "fighting a cold." When congestion and cough arrive, it is now dubbed a "miserable cold." After a few days of "nursing a cold," we reach the "tail end of a cold."

Symptoms of a Cold

You might feel a bit unwell or have a slight chilling sensation. This is your first sign that you could be coming down with a cold. Perhaps this chilling sensation contributed to the idea that colds are caused by cold weather.

The cardinal symptoms of a cold are sneezing, stuffy nose, a scratchy, sore throat, and a cough. A slight fever, but no higher than 101 degrees Fahrenheit, is common. Sneezing, nasal discharge, and congestion begin on the first day and rapidly increase in severity by the second or third day. A cough and hoarseness may begin early in the illness and, if they do, tend to persist until the end of the symptoms. Some people complain of a loss of their sense of smell or taste or a feeling of pressure in their ears or sinuses, and their voice becomes nasal or hoarse due to the inflammation of the vocal cords by the virus.

Causes of Colds

The eight different groups of cold viruses include over two hundred different varieties. While you will develop immunity to a given virus after recovering from a cold, that leaves 199 other viruses that can cause you to sneeze and cough. About half of all cold viruses are in the *rhinovirus* group, named after the Greek word for "nose." A form of the rhinovirus was the first cold virus identified, in the early 1950s. The more than one hundred types of rhino viruses cause problems year-round and are particularly prevalent in the late summer and early autumn. It is not a coincidence that this period coincides with the start of the school year. Not only does the rhinovirus like this season, but the school year provides countless opportunities for it to grow as millions of children are crowded together inside classrooms.

The second most frequent cause of colds are the *coronaviruses*. Discovered in 1965, they're named after the crownlike extensions that surround them. Coronaviruses are spread by airborne droplets from coughs and sneezes and tend to strike in midwinter. A form of the coronavirus caused SARS in China, a fatal, coldlike illness that spread around the world, ultimately taking three thousand lives in 2002.

The Other Cold Viruses

The *respiratory syncytial virus* (RSV) is round with protruding spikes and strikes in deep winter. It affects the lower respiratory tract and is most often a problem for children and infants.

Parainfluenza viruses are the largest of all cold viruses. They cause colds in infants and children that can lead to croup, bronchiolitis, and pneumonia.

The *Coxsackie virus* looks like an eight-sided crystal and was named after Coxsackie, New York, where it first made two hundred people sick with a bad cough and fever.

The *adenovirus* is an artistic structure of facets and knob-tipped rods. It produces colds in late winter, spring, and early summer—often causing those summer colds where you can't figure out if it's an allergy or a cold. It rarely affects people over

SARS: THE COLD THAT KILLS

In November 2002, a new, severe respiratory disease broke out in the south-China province of Guangdong. In just six weeks, it spread to every continent on the globe. Named severe adult respiratory syndrome (SARS), it starts with flulike symptoms of fever, cough, and body aches. Within three to five days, just when a flu should start to be loosening its grip, SARS victims become acutely ill. The lungs fill with fluid, fever soars, and the kidneys begin to fail. In people over age sixty-five, death rates hover around 50 percent.

The cause of SARS is a new, deadly strain of the common corona cold virus. These spiked viruses normally cause disease in animals, and a mild disease in humans. The coronavirus that causes SARS originated in civet cats sold in the live-animal food markets in rural China. Doctors now know that the first cases of SARS occurred in people who handled these cats in the open-air markets. Then in a shift in pattern that shocked public health officials around the world, the first SARS victims were able to spread the disease directly to their family, neighbors, and health care workers in the hospitals where they went for help. Highly contagious, a single SARS patient could infect dozens of doctors and nurses caring for him. By the time the epidemic had been brought under control, eight thousand people had become ill and eight hundred had died.

With the start of warm, sunny weather in the spring of 2002, SARS, like other cold-weather illnesses, seemed to fade away. During the summer doctors watched anxiously for signs that SARS would reappear again with the other seasonal colds and flus. To lower chances of recurrence, Chinese health officials eliminated the civet cats that harbored the virus and instituted new restrictions on the handling and housing of animals. To date, the international vigilance has worked. SARS has remained rare and isolated, limited to people working with animals in Southeast Asia.

age fifteen and in adults produces mild, often undetectable illness.

The *echovirus,* close cousin of the Coxsackie virus, causes colds with fever, sore throat, and a particularly severe cough.

Transmission of Colds

Not only are there over two hundred cold viruses, but they can be transmitted in a number of ways. The rhinovirus is spread through direct contact. That is, if you shake hands with somebody who has a cold, and then touch your face, this contact can transmit virus-laden mucus from one person to another. You can also pick up a rhinovirus by contact with fomites—inanimate objects such as doorknobs or pens. Cold viruses can live for hours on handrails, tissues, even telephones. When you handle them, you will transmit the virus to your fingers, and when you touch your face, eyes, or nose, it gets directly into your mucosal tissues.

Other viruses, such as the coronavirus, are spread in the air, through virus-laden droplets. When an infected person sneezes or coughs, these droplets fill the air. When they are inhaled by others, they can spread the infection.

Impact of Infection

The cold virus first settles into the nose and starts replicating in the cells of the upper airways. The cold virus has a somewhat unusual way of causing disease in the body. Once most viruses get into a body, they enter cells, replicate, then thousands of newly formed viruses burst out of the dead cell. By contrast, most cold viruses don't destroy cells. They enter the cells and reproduce, but the cells remain whole and alive. Cold viruses cause symptoms because their presence provokes the body to produce inflammatory compounds called kinins or mediators, including prostaglandins and histamine. Bradykinin and the

COLD AND FLU OLD WIVES' TALE #1: KISSING CAUSES COLDS

With colds, just about the safest contact is kissing, because few or no cold viruses are in saliva. Fluid from the nose or the eyes has virus. But simply kissing somebody will usually not spread the cold. How many times have people said to you, "I can't kiss you because I have a cold"? Well, that's not the problem.

leukotrienes are mediators that create aches and pains throughout the body. These chemicals are a protective mechanism, but they're not that helpful, and they produce unpleasant symptoms.

One major impact of these chemicals is swelling inside the airways. Cytokine-provoked inflammation causes the blood vessels to leak fluid. There is an increase in mucus as white blood cells rush to attack the invading viruses, releasing even more irritating compounds, causing you to feel even more congested. Histamine cause sneezing, and the prostaglandins produce fever. Cough develops as a result of the bronchial irritation of the excess mucus that's produced during the cold.

Many colds occur in the winter, which gives rise to the idea that cold weather causes colds. Actually, the weather has more to do with the preference of the virus than the impact of frosty weather on your health or resistance. Many cold viruses thrive in colder temperatures. Researchers have done some pretty extreme experiments to study the role of weather on colds. Volunteers were hosed down with cold water, left to walk around outside in the cold, and then watched to see if they developed a cold. They didn't. A control group was then inoculated with a cold virus and kept warm and comfortable in a dorm room. Most of those inoculated did come down with sniffles and sneezes.

COLD AND FLU OLD WIVES' TALE #2:
COLD WEATHER CAN GIVE YOU
A COLD

Some experiments suggest that the stress of being cold and wet can lower your immunity and lead to a cold, but temperature alone is not a factor.

Diagnosis of a Cold

We rarely do laboratory or viral testing to confirm the diagnosis of a cold and, for the most part, diagnose on the basis of symptoms and examination. It's not a hard diagnosis to make. What's important is to differentiate a cold from the other respiratory infections such as acute bronchitis, pneumonia, or even influenza, because the treatment for each is different and different complications can develop.

If new symptoms and problems develop during a cold, then we can use more sophisticated diagnostic techniques. For example, if you develop continuing pain around the eyes, I will suspect that a sinus infection has settled in. To make a better diagnosis, I might send you for sinus X-rays to confirm an infection in these easily congested hollow bones. If a cough continues for more than two weeks and perhaps you complain of chest pain when you take a deep breath, I would call for a chest X-ray to rule out pneumonia. But if you are under age fifty and have no underlying health problems, it is not necessary to do expensive testing when the problem seems contained and self-limiting.

Complications of Colds

A cold is generally considered a nuisance disease, but complications are not uncommon. The standard cold has a five-to-seven-

THE DIFFERENCE BETWEEN A COLD AND AN ALLERGY

First, consider the season. If symptoms strike during the school year from September to March, the culprit is more likely to be a virus. Allergies can strike year-round and are especially common in the spring and summer. Colds develop slowly over a day or two, cause a bit of fever, usually affect more than one person in a home, school, or workplace, and last five to seven days. Allergies come on quickly and can last as little as a few hours and do not cause fever. If you are the only one coughing and sneezing at home or work, it's likely to be an allergy rather than a contagious virus.

day course: by the end of a week, all symptoms are pretty much gone. But that's a normal progression. About 25 percent of even uncomplicated colds can last for two weeks. A sign that a cold has taken a bad turn would be that the cold seems to be getting better after a few days, then seems to be getting worse. You develop a higher fever, the cough gets worse, and you genuinely feel sicker. This is definitely a signal to call your physician.

About 80 percent of people with colds develop some degree of sinusitis, which is an infection in the sinuses. After a week of sneezing and coughing, instead of cold symptoms starting to fade, new problems arise. Pain around the eyes, a rise in fever, and an increase in congestion could signal that the cold has led to a bacterial infection of the sinuses. Chapter 5 offers a full discussion on recognizing and treating sinus problems.

Secondary bronchitis can also develop alongside colds, and up to 60 percent of cold sufferers develop some degree of problem in the lower airways. A cough that just refuses to go away is a sign that bronchitis has developed. It is such a common problem that chapter 6 is devoted to recognizing and treating it.

People frequently consult with me about a lingering cold,

concerned that they have developed pneumonia. While fewer than .3 percent of people with colds go on to develop pneumonia, this serious respiratory infection needs aggressive medical attention. Pneumonia usually occurs only when there are other factors such as age or underlying health problems. In the very young, a cold can develop into a serious pulmonary problem, such as croup, bronchiolitis, or pneumonia. For the elderly, pneumonia can be sudden and fatal. Pneumonia and influenza combined are the sixth leading cause of death in the United States, and over 90 percent of people who die of pneumonia are elderly. Over thirty different forms of pneumonia exist, and we're going to be talking about them in chapter 8.

We don't fully understand why complications occur, but we know some factors that increase the risk of developing more serious health problems. Lowered immunity can allow a cold to turn into something more serious. As we grow older, our ability to mount a defense against infection declines, making us more vulnerable to disease. For example, the flu vaccine is 70–80 percent effective for children and adults—yet by the time you reach age seventy, the vaccine is only 40 percent effective. National statistics from the CDC show that 90 percent of people hospitalized for pneumonia are over sixty-five.

Underlying health problems can increase your risk for complications. If you are diabetic, the higher blood sugar levels raise the chance that a viral infection can develop into bacterial sinusitis or bronchitis.

The irritable airways of an asthmatic are also more likely to become superinfected with bacteria. Additionally, a simple viral infection can trigger a full-blown asthma attack.

Complications can arise even in young, healthy people, when a particularly virulent strain of virus causes a respiratory infection. The recent avian flu virus produced a rapidly progressing pneumonia that was fatal to three out of four victims.

Rather than becoming frightened that every sniffle could be the start of a deadly pneumonia, by understanding the dynamics of both normal disease as well as potential complications, you can recognize early signs to keep problems small and manageable—or even avoid them entirely.

Immunity to Colds

Because there are so many cold viruses, we have to develop resistance to different ones. Children get six to eight colds a year. As we grow older and leave school, we get fewer colds. The incidence of colds jumps when adults start their own family: during these years you may get almost as many colds as your children. Mothers seem to have a higher rate of catching colds than fathers. Fathers have the lowest rate of infection of anybody in the family. Then the number of colds decreases as your children grow older and leave home. There is another spurt of colds when your children have grandchildren: you, in taking care of them, will contract colds. But in general, as you grow older, you have fewer colds per year. Doctors suspect that we've actually acquired immunity to at least several dozen different viruses, so that when a virus attacks, your body says, "Oh! I've seen this one before," and pumps out the specific antibody to the virus.

COLDS AND FLU OLD WIVES' TALE #3: YOU'RE NOT CONTAGIOUS WITHOUT A FEVER

Since most colds have very little fever, this is a poor indication of your risk to others. Children can actually spread a cold up to two days before they develop a single sniffle. Adults are most contagious at the height of their sneezing and coughing, but will continue to shed virus (albeit in lower numbers) for the duration of the seven days of active infection.

The Geography of Colds

Colds happen worldwide. They happen in the Arctic, and they happen in tropical regions. Different areas have different cold seasons. In temperate climates like that of the United States, the cold season begins in late August and September. The number of people with colds rises sharply for a few weeks and remains elevated until early spring. During April and May, cold rates level off, then drop to low summertime levels.

In tropical areas, the cold season corresponds to the rainy season. Researchers also speculate that the winter and rainy months are also a time when people stay indoors. The windows are closed. There's less exchange of air, and there's greater chance for person-to-person contagion.

Cigarette smokers, interestingly, have the same number of colds as nonsmokers, but their colds are more severe. For people with asthma, colds can trigger asthmatic attacks, and colds should be viewed much more seriously by most people with asthma than by generally healthy individuals at any age. Colds in people with underlying lung problems such as chronic bronchitis or emphysema can trigger an exacerbation. I tell my pulmonary patients to call me at the first sign of a cold because we want to pay close attention to its progression and take action if the cough or fever become pronounced or prolonged.

Preventing a Cold

In my first year of medical school when we went on the wards, we got a pep talk by the infectious-disease consult: "There are three rules for preventing infectious disease. One, wash your hands. Two, wash your hands. And three, wash your hands." This is certainly true of colds. Simply washing your hands with soap and water has been shown to significantly decrease the spread of colds. In a Toronto study, students were asked to keep a log of the number of times they washed their hands and

THE TIME OF THE MONTH FOR COLDS

Women experience an increased number of colds in the midpoint of their menstrual cycle. Doctors suspect that this is a time when immunity seems to drop.

the incidence of cold symptoms. The result? Those who washed their hands more than seven times a day had more than four times *fewer* colds than those who soaped up less frequently. Remember that rhinoviruses, which produce half of all colds, are spread primarily by direct contact.

It is not necessary to use antibacterial soap, since its chemicals don't affect the cold virus. However, solutions of alcohol-based hand sanitizers and sprays such as Lysol have been shown to be anti-microbial—that is, they can kill both viruses and bacteria. During the cold season, it's a good idea to wipe down the bathrooms and your kitchen countertops with these types of sanitizing cleansers to control the cold viruses in your own home.

When a cold strikes in a home, using disposable tissues and getting rid of them in a plastic bag will also help contain the spread of cold virus inside the house.

DON'T LEND OR BORROW PENS

Each time you go to a restaurant or store and make a purchase on your credit card, you're offered a pen when you're given your charge receipt. During the flu season, this pen is passed to dozens of people each day and is a superb carrier of cold viruses. Simply by using your own pen and not lending it out, you can significantly cut down on your exposure to the cold virus. Remember, use your own pen to sign for packages, credit slips, and to sign in at the doctor's office.

"OLD-TIME" HOME REMEDIES FOR COLDS

- Eat garlic
- Don't eat garlic
- Get some sunshine
- Rub socks with onions
- Avoid wheat
- Sniff cinnamon
- Grow a thick mustache
- Stand on your head

Treatment Issues for Colds

Like my patient Mrs. Salazar, we are all frustrated that there is no cure for an illness as simple as a cold. Since there is no shot or pill to banish the cold bug, we need to address the symptoms. Yet doctors tend to ignore cold symptoms. They know that colds are not life-threatening and feel confident that you will soon be well. It is left to the patient to come up with solutions for symptom relief. A seemingly endless assortment of pills, sprays, and syrups are offered to treat colds. The trick is to know which ones to use and how to take them.

We know that much of the discomfort of a cold is due to the release of inflammatory cytokines in reaction to the presence of the cold virus, and we have the tools to reduce the release of these irritants. We can use aspirin, acetaminophen such as Tylenol, and ibuprofen such as Advil to block prostaglandins, which provoke fever and headache. Antihistamines block the mediators that cause blood vessels to leak fluid leading to congestion. Decongestants act by shrinking blood vessels, allowing air and mucus to move more freely in the nose and sinuses.

Hot fluids like tea and chicken soup thin mucus congestion

TREATMENT PLAN: COLDS

ANTIHISTAMINE

- Antihistamine twice a day. If you can sleep during the day, use a traditional antihistamine in the morning. If you need to be alert during the day, use a traditional product only at night.

DECONGESTANT

- If you are using a nasal-spray decongestant, switch to an oral preparation after three days.
- Use a decongestant as directed by manufacturer.

ANTI-INFLAMMATORY

- Take acetaminophen, aspirin, or ibuprofen every four hours for the first three or four days of a cold. Reduce to twice a day for the next three days.

QUELLING THE COUGH

- Start with cough drops that contain soothing ingredients such as honey and throat-numbing ingredients such as benzocaine.
- If cough persists, use cough syrup with dextromethorphan.

ANTIBIOTICS

- Not necessary for a simple cold. However, if you have asthma or COPD, antibiotics may be prescribed to avoid a flare-up of breathing problems due to secondary bacterial infection.

and allow the upper airways to drain. In addition, research from the University of Nebraska has demonstrated that hot chicken soup can block the production of inflammatory cells called neutrophils.

Vaccines

- None available for colds.

Antiviral Drugs

- None commercially available for colds.

Nutritional Therapy

- Chicken soup one or two times a day for the first three days of symptoms.
- Daily glass of orange juice.
- Three to four cups hot tea daily.
- Additional fluids: diet ginger ale, iced tea, cold water.
- Light meals for the first three to four days, then regular meal plan.

Hydrotherapy

- Relieve nasal congestion with saline rinse two to three times a day.
- Relieve throat pain with saline gargle twice a day.
- Hot showers in the morning to loosen mucus in airways.
- If congested at night, use steam inhaler for three to five minutes before going to sleep.

Supplements

- Zinc spray every two to three hours at first sign of a cold.
- Zinc lozenges to relieve sore throat pain.
- Up to 500 mg of vitamin C daily for up to seven days after cold symptoms first appear.

CHAPTER 5

SINUSITIS—THE COLD
THAT LINGERS

Mrs. Glazer tended to worry. She worried that the wax on her cucumbers could increase her risk of developing cancer. When the weather was hot, she worried that it was a sign that the hole in the ozone layer was growing; and when she developed a lingering headache, she was convinced it was a sign of a brain tumor. After a short history and examination, I was happy to tell her that her pain was not due to a fatal brain tumor. Mrs. Glazer had acute sinusitis.

Mrs. Glazer is in good company. According to the Centers for Disease Control and Prevention, each year sinus problems affect 37 million Americans, are responsible for 18 million doctor office visits, and cost more than $6 billion in health care. A survey from the National Center for Health Statistics found that sinus problems are responsible for 13 million lost workdays and 2 million school absences.

Sinusitis is an inflammation of the sinus cavities that surround the face. The four pairs of symmetrical sinus cavities include the *frontal* sinus (just above the eyes), the *maxillary* sinus (over the cheek), the *ethmoid* sinus (along the nose), and the *sphenoid* sinuses (behind the nose) (See Illustration on page 76). The sinuses are covered by the same mucous membrane that coats the upper airway. The mucus that forms inside these sinuses is brushed out two to three times a day as a result of the motion of the cilia inside the sinuses. However, the drainage passages that connect the sinuses to the nasal pharynx are narrow. If they become inflamed because of a viral or bacterial infection or an allergy, mucus backs up into the sinuses. Since the mucus, acting like flypaper, collects bacteria and other organisms, these can multiply and cause an infection in the sinuses.

Doctors classify sinusitis as either acute or chronic.

ACUTE SINUSITIS

Symptoms of Acute Sinusitis

The symptoms of acute sinusitis can include a stuffy, runny nose, toothache, a loss of smell and taste, cough, headache, pain around the eyes and cheeks, and a sense of pressure when bending forward. They can vary from mild and annoying to severe and disabling. Sinusitis is considered acute if the symptoms have been present less than six weeks.

Causes of Acute Sinusitis

Acute sinusitis is primarily the result of colds, frequently caused by bacteria, and occasionally linked to fungi. Far and away the most common cause of acute sinusitis is a viral infection. When you get a cold, the sinuses are almost always involved. Viruses spread through the various openings that connect the sinuses to the nose and to the pharynx. In fact, about half of all colds include some degree of sinusitis.

The second most common cause of sinusitis are bacteria. It

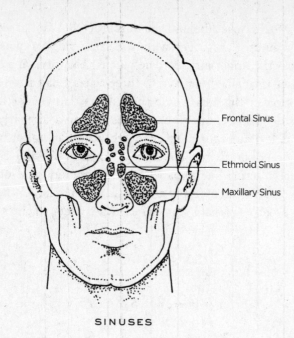

Frontal Sinus

Ethmoid Sinus

Maxillary Sinus

SINUSES

is estimated that out of the 1 billion colds that Americans get each year, up to 2 percent of these become secondarily infected with bacteria, resulting in acute bacterial sinusitis. That amounts to about 20 million cases of bacterial sinusitis each year.

Although colds due to the rhinovirus almost invariably result in some degree of sinusitis, the sinuses can also become infected with bacteria that normally live harmlessly in our upper airways. These organisms, such as streptococcus and *Haemophilus influenzae,* are routinely eliminated as the cilia sweep away the mucus in regular cleaning of the airway. But when obstruction occurs, as with a common cold, they accumulate and cannot effectively be removed. Keep in mind your sinuses don't become infected from somebody else's bacteria. They become infected by your own bacteria.

Diagnosis of Acute Sinusitis

No one would be surprised to hear a cold sufferer say, "My head aches and I feel congested." What is probably less well-known is that these are also signs of acute sinusitis. The majority of people who have colds also have acute viral sinusitis. Most colds disappear within seven to ten days. Colds that linger beyond that, or new symptoms such as high fever and cloudy mucus that develop late in the duration of the cold, suggest acute bacterial sinusitis.

X-rays and CT scans can demonstrate obstruction of the sinuses and may even suggest what type of sinusitis is causing problems. On an X-ray, substances that are dense (such as bone) appear white. Structures that are thin (such as air) appear black. Normally sinuses are filled with air and appear black on X-rays, while the solid bones of the skull appear white or opaque.

When a sinus becomes obstructed, it can fill up entirely with mucus and become totally white on an X-ray. A partially filled sinus shows what is called an "air fluid level" on an X-ray: the part of the sinus that has accumulations of mucus looks white; the area above the fluid still appears black. Keep in mind that X-ray findings may not be able to differentiate between viral or bacterial sinusitis. They simply show disease in the sinus, but not necessarily the actual type.

A simple test that gives some of the same information as the more complicated X-rays and CT scans is called *transillumination*. To perform this test, I turn off the lights in the room, place a small, lit flashlight firmly against the skin just underneath your eye, and look for an illumination in the maxillary sinus. I can also ask you to open your mouth, and looking up at the palate, I will see if the light shines through. If it doesn't shine through, it is equivalent to finding an *opacified* or fluid-filled sinus on an X-ray.

IS IT SINUSITIS OR A MIGRAINE?

The symptoms are so familiar—recurrent, long-lasting pain and pressure around the eyes and discomfort when bending over. But these are not necessarily sinus problems. Doctors suspect that a similarity in the type and pattern of symptoms to migraine has frequently led to misdiagnosis and the wrong treatment choices. In a study released by the National Headache Foundation, out of thirty patients with suspected sinus problems, twenty-nine actually had migraines. A good way to separate the two problems? Try one of the instant-dissolve serotonin inhibitors such as Imitrex or Maxalt developed specifically for migraines. If the problem is due to migraine swelling of the blood vessels rather than clogged sinuses, the relief will be rapid and dramatic.

The Question of a Culture

With bacterial pneumonia and strep throat we can easily take samples to try to identify the offending organisms. Unfortunately it is much more difficult to culture material from your sinus. A swab of the the inside of your nose is not a representative sample for bacteria that might be causing problems in your sinus cavities. A sinus culture requires that a needle puncture the sinus. As you are probably wincing from just this description, you can imagine that this maneuver is rarely performed. It is sometimes done in clinical studies to demonstrate the effectiveness of an antibiotic, but even in these circumstances it is uncommon. Diagnosis is therefore done on the basis of symptoms, X-rays, and your response to treatment. Because we may not know if the acute sinusitis is caused by a virus or bacteria, much less what type of bacteria we are dealing with, treating acute sinusitis means developing a working relationship with your doctor.

Treatment Issues

Relieving acute sinusitis starts with cleaning clogged air passages by rinsing the nostrils with a mild saline solution. These are available commercially, or you can make your own by combining one heaping teaspoon of kosher salt, one-half teaspoon of baking soda, and one pint of warm water. First blow your nose gently before spraying. With your head upright, spray the medicine once into each nostril, sniffing while squeezing the bottle quickly and firmly. Wait three to five minutes to allow the drug to work, then blow your nose gently again. A total of two to three sprays should be administered at each dosing. Keep the spray bottle at room temperature and away from direct heat or light.

Decongestants will help to dissolve and mobilize even dry, hardened mucus, opening airways to improve breathing. Don't blow vigorously. Although it will clear nasal passages momentarily, the strong pressure that occurs within the nasal passage as you blow against a blocked nasal outlet pushes bacteria that are normally in the nasal pharynx deep into the sinuses—sharply increasing chances of bacterial sinusitis.

Decongestant spray will shrink swollen membranes to provide further, albeit temporary, relief. Acute bacterial sinusitis needs additional antibiotic therapy. I start by prescribing five to seven days of a broad-spectrum antibiotic such as Augmentin, since I don't really know which organism is causing the infection. If symptoms do not improve within forty-eight hours, I will switch to another antibiotic such Levaquin, a fluoroquinolone.

Prevention of Acute Sinusitis

Preventing acute sinusitis starts by taking steps to avoid the cold virus that provokes the problems in your airways. Wash hands frequently, avoid using public phones, and don't borrow

TREATMENT PLAN:
ACUTE BACTERIAL SINUSITIS

ANTIHISTAMINE

- Antihistamine not helpful. May actually thicken mucus in nasal passages and prolong infection.

DECONGESTANT

- Phenylephrine spray for three to four days.
- If symptoms persist, use a systemic decongestant in pill or liquid form.

ANTI-INFLAMMATORY

- Use acetaminophen, ibuprofen, or aspirin one to two times per day if headache pain is present.

COUGH CONTROL

- Not required.

ANTIBIOTICS

- First-line therapy—Amoxicillin, Augmentin, Bactrim, for seven days.
- Second-line therapy (if allergic to penicillin and/or sulfa drugs)—Levaquin for seven days.

VACCINES

- None available.

ANTIVIRAL DRUGS

- Not applicable.

NUTRITIONAL THERAPY

- Regular meals, prepared with lower salt.
- Chicken soup once a day.
- Three to four cups hot tea daily.
- Spicy tomato juice.

HYDROTHERAPY

- Hot shower in a.m.
- Saline nasal spray three times a day.

SUPPLEMENTS

- None specifically indicated.

or lend pens. If you seem to develop colds frequently, avoid shaking hands. When you are exposed to people with colds, use a zinc nasal spray to discourage viral growth. While there is conflicting data on zinc and colds, in the laboratory zinc gluconate can stop cold viruses from replicating.

When colds develop, hot drinks and hot showers will thin out virus-induced mucus. This will lower fluid buildup in the airways that will block sinus drainage.

Complications of Acute Sinusitis

By and large most acute sinusitis is a mild disease, just like the common cold—because it is part of the common cold. However, complications of acute bacterial sinusitis are much more ominous. Fortunately they affect a small minority of patients who have bacterial sinusitis, but since they can be life-threatening, these complications are one of the reasons why doctors, when they diagnose acute bacterial sinusitis, are not reluctant to use

FLY EASY

Research has shown that 20 percent of airline passengers develop colds within a week of their flight. To decrease your risk of respiratory infections, try using zinc nasal spray before and after a flight.

antibiotics. Although there has been a great push to reduce the use of antibiotics, it would appear that in the case of acute bacterial sinusitis, they are still indicated.

Most of the complications are caused by direct extension of the sinus infection to other parts of the head. One of the more frequent complications is the spread of the infection to the eye area. Called *orbital cellulitis,* it can be a potentially serious problem and can cause permanent blindness in up to 10 percent of cases. Symptoms include swelling, redness, and pain around the eye. The eye is painful and difficult to move, and double vision is common. Diagnosis is made by physical examination, and treatment consists of broad-spectrum antibiotics usually administered in a hospital. Surgery may be required to remove infected material to save the eye.

When the organisms that are causing problems in the sinus spread to the neighboring bones, the result is called *osteomyelitis.* There are usually few symptoms and the infection is diagnosed when a CT scan is taken to check on a sinus infection that has failed to respond to treatment. The scan will show a fluid-filled space that may also contain fragments of destroyed bone. Osteomyelitis is treated with intravenous antibiotics and occasionally surgery.

When a sinus infection leads to meningitis, an infection of the superficial membrane that coats the brain and the spinal cord, the symptoms are clear and dramatic: severe headache, rise in fever, stiff neck, confusion, and extreme fatigue. If untreated, this form of meningitis can rapidly be fatal. Diagnosis is confirmed by a spinal tap, which shows an increase in white blood cells and a low sugar level. The immediate infection is treated with intravenous antibiotics, but surgery may be needed to remove obstructions in the sinus that led to the infection of the spinal cord.

Sinus infections can also spread to a large vein in the eye area. Called the *cavernous sinus,* it can develop blood clots as a response to infection. Symptoms begin with a headache so severe patients seek immediate medical attention. Spiking high fever soon develops, followed by swelling in the eye area, and the muscles that move the eye may become partially paralyzed. For an accurate diagnosis, a contrast CT scan is needed. A dye, injected into a vein, travels to the eye area and outlines the cavernous sinus, showing the clot and the infection. The mainstay of treatment is high-dose intravenous antibiotics. Anticoagulants (drugs that thin the blood), steroids to reduce inflammation, and surgery may be needed.

One of the most feared complications of sinusitis is the brain abscess, in which the infection spreads to the brain, where it causes a localized, walled-off infection, much like a large boil deep inside the brain. The abscess has properties of both an infection and a tumor, causing both pressure and destruction of brain tissue. Symptoms can start insidiously with headache and blurred or double vision. At other times a brain abscess can announce its presence dramatically with seizures or a stroke. Diagnosed with a CT scan and spinal tap, it can successfully be treated with a combination of antibiotics and surgery to remove the abscess.

The incidence of these troubling but relatively uncommon complications has declined since the advent of antibiotics. Although all doctors are concerned about the rise of bacteria that are resistant to antibiotics, the prospect of these serious problems makes the right choice of antibiotics important for the treatment of acute bacterial sinusitis.

CHRONIC SINUSITIS

Chronic sinusitis is simply defined as a sinus condition that continues for at least six weeks to three months. If you have sinus problems, that definition just doesn't do the problem justice. Chronic sinusitis is that cold that starts at Thanksgiving and stays with you until the spring thaw. It is the headache that pounds for weeks or a toothache that has you wishing for novocaine. Sometimes it gets better, sometimes it gets worse, but it is never really gone.

Despite its widespread occurrence, nobody truly understands the dynamics of chronic sinusitis. Some experts believe that chronic sinusitis is the result of acute bacterial sinusitis that is inadequately treated or is treated so that the infection and inflammation are not caught in time. As a result, obstruction remains, and the sinuses become damaged in such a way that they are prone to recurring episodes of sinusitis.

There is a strong relationship between chronic sinusitis and allergies. Studies have shown that up to 80 percent of all people with chronic sinusitis have allergies. Plants, pets, molds, even cold air, can trigger an allergic reaction that creates a virtual war in the airways.

Allergists frequently view chronic sinusitis as "asthma of the upper airways." Up to 65 percent of people with asthma also have chronic sinusitis. These doctors point out that both the upper airways (the nose and throat) and lower airways (trachea and lungs) have similar mucous membranes. Researchers have also found similar types of inflammatory cells and compounds in the noses of people with chronic sinusitis as are found in the lungs of people with asthma. In addition, it has been shown that treating sinusitis improves asthma.

Symptoms of Chronic Sinusitis

The symptoms of chronic sinusitis may vary from a mild, occasional congestion to the same symptoms as acute rhinitis, but not as dramatic. Patients with chronic sinusitis may complain of pain over the sinus area, discomfort in their teeth, and a chronic sense of congestion in their nose and head. From time to time these are punctuated by acute episodes where the sinuses may become infected with bacteria.

Impact of Infection

The sinuses seem designed to fail. They have extremely narrow passages that curve and twist. At some points, the drainage actually calls for the fluids to go upward, against the pull of gravity. It is suspected that some individuals have especially narrow or twisted sinus passages and are anatomically destined to have upper airway problems.

Keep in mind that cigarette smoke paralyzes the housekeeping activity of the cilia inside the nose. Not surprisingly, regular smoking has been linked to an increase in sinus problems.

Chronic sinusitis provokes and is then worsened by the development of nasal polyps. These are fleshy, noncancerous outgrowths from the mucus membranes inside the nose. They form around the tiny sinus openings, making both drainage of mucus as well as breathing much more difficult.

Polyps tend to develop during infections, allergies, or even long-term exposure to irritating chemicals. It's not uncommon for people with asthma to develop nasal polyps. Over time, polyps tend to grow, shrink, then grow again. Even if you have them surgically removed, if you tend to develop polyps, they can recur.

Ear, nose, and throat (ENT) specialists judge the size and

extent of the polyps and treat them with medication or remove them surgically.

Diagnosis of Chronic Sinusitis

Diagnosing chronic sinusitis primarily entails understanding the definition of this disease. Chronic sinusitis is acute sinusitis that doesn't resolve after six weeks to three months. The symptoms may be similar to those of acute sinusitis, although generally they are less severe and maybe punctuated from time to time with bouts of acute sinusitis. A physician consulted by someone with chronic sinusitis should probably obtain sinus X-rays, a CT scan of the skull, or an MRI.

The CT scan is a form of X-ray that allows the interior of the body to be viewed in a three-dimensional perspective. Instead of presenting the skull as a flat surface, a CT scan allows us to cut through the image in successive slices. This allows us to see all the air, tissue spaces, and bones individually in the sinus cavities. It allows us to define anatomy more accurately, providing a virtual road map of the problems in the upper airways. If surgery is being considered, it lets us see if it is truly needed and tells us if repair is possible.

In patients who have chronic sinus conditions, the fluid may have resorbed or may have drained to an extent, but what is left behind is a thickened mucosal surface. In other words, the surface covering of the sinuses is thickened and more dense. We call this *remodeling* of the tissues, and it will show up clearly on a CT. This remodeling is a consequence of the chronic inflammation and consists of scarred, damaged, and dysfunctional tissue covering the walls of the sinuses. The remodeled tissue does not clear out bacteria and toxin-rich mucus, so that the upper airways are permanently obstructed and are more likely to become reinfected with bacteria or viruses.

Complications of Chronic Sinusitis

As you can imagine, once the sinuses are damaged by the presence of chronic inflammation, they are much more likely—even in the absence of an acute infection with a virus—to develop an obstruction, and as a result develop acute bacterial sinusitis. It is not uncommon for acute bacterial sinusitis to complicate the picture of chronic sinusitis. Repeated bouts of acute bacterial sinusitis in someone with chronic sinus symptoms indicate, again, the need for specialized X-rays and referral to an ear, nose, and throat specialist.

In recent years we have become aware that nasal fungus can cause chronic sinusitis. In addition to traditional symptoms, fungal sinusitis can produce foul-smelling mucus or extremely bad breath because the fungus is actually destroying sinus tissue.

An advanced imaging technique called *magnetic resonance* imaging or MRI can assist with the diagnosis of fungal sinusitis. MRI does not use radiation to explore the body. It combines a large magnet, a radio-wave transmitter, and a computer to provide detailed pictures of bones and blood vessels. The MRI scans your body with a magnetic field and bursts of radio waves. In reaction, your body emits signals that are picked up and sent to a computer, which projects an image of the body's structures. With an MRI I can see tiny changes in the structures of the tissues.

In an MRI image, body parts with a high water content (e.g., fatty tissue) appear light, while drier parts (e.g., bones) appear dark. The MRI can even produce clear images of organs that are surrounded by bones, so it is an ideal tool to examine the brain and face.

Fungal growth appears black on the MRI, while bacterial or allergic sinusitis appears white. New forms of aerosolized drugs are now available for treatment of this condition. Medications including amphotericin and fluconazole are inhaled through the nose via a device called a nebulizer, which produces a fine mist of medication. It provides better delivery of the drug to the affected sinuses and as a bonus causes fewer side effects, such as stomach upset and fatigue, compared to medication that has to be swallowed or given intravenously.

In the invasive form of fungal sinusitis, the disease is dramatic. It can cause shock and high fevers and invade the bloodstream, and people can succumb rapidly, though this is extremely unusual. With the more chronic "indolent" form of the disease, a fungus ball forms within the sinus. A fungal sinus infection in an otherwise healthy individual is frequently difficult to distinguish from chronic sinusitis and its acute exacerbations. As a result of chronic fungal sinusitis, the draining passages can become blocked, and bacteria can overgrow and cause secondary acute exacerbations of this chronic condition.

Treatment Issues of Acute Bacterial Sinusitis

Treatment of acute bacterial sinusitis is usually seven to ten days of older, narrow-spectrum antibiotics. When the infection becomes chronic, the treatment usually calls for three to six weeks of newer antibiotics such as Augmentin, which combines amoxicillin and clavulanic acid, or a newer broad-spectrum antibiotic such as Levaquin. With chronic sinusitis,

---

SINUS QUICK TIP:
HUM AWAY SINUS PAIN

According to a recent study out of Sweden, humming a few bars of your favorite tune can lower risk of developing sinusitis. Researchers found that humming increases ventilation of the sinus cavities and increases air exchange within the hollow bones in the skull.

the organism involved may be resistant, so the choice and timing of the antibiotic treatment has to address this problem. Newer antibiotics are more likely to be effective against resistant bacteria. However, using the newer antibiotics indiscriminately will lead to the early emergence of bacterial resistance to them. Current practice and guidelines are to reserve the newer agents for more difficult situations, and those situations in which the bacteria are probably resistant to older antibiotics.

Treatment Issues in Chronic Sinusitis

Decongestants, which can provide relief in acute forms of sinusitis, are not as helpful for chronic sinusitis. Decongestant sprays that directly shrink swollen airways can only be used for three days in a row so as to avoid the problem of rebound congestion. As the spray wears off, the small blood vessels expand again, producing feelings of congestion. The returning symptoms are so unpleasant, you spray again. This can actually lead to a drug dependency that can persist for years. Patients with this problem must often work with an ENT specialist to go through decongestant withdrawal.

Medications to control the allergies that can cause infected sinuses may offer help in addition to the tried-and-true antihistamines. We now have new agents that block the development of other allergy provokers, such leukotrienes, which when released by the body cause the airways to constrict and increase mucus production. Leukotriene inhibitors such as Singulair have been shown to be effective against allergies. Mast cells are allergy-causing factories, producing both leukotrienes and histamines. These cells, distributed throughout the body, are felt to help regulate the inflammatory response. As with other agents of this response, unusual environmental stresses or genetic predispositions can bring about imbalances, causing illness such as allergy. A mast cell stabilizer called Intal has provided relief in cases where other medications have failed.

The inflammation of chronic sinusitis can persist long after the infection or allergic reaction has been brought under control. Anti-inflammatory agents such as inhaled steroids can prevent the cascade of irritating agents that are released in an infection or allergic reaction. Products such as Flonase or Rhinocort, which contain steroids, are sprayed into the nose to reduce inflammation, swelling, and discomfort.

When treating chronic sinusitis, the physician is always aware that the medical management of this disease may be disappointing, because this is not simply a disease of infection, but also one of altered anatomy. Because of the chronic damage that has been done to the sinus passages and to the sinuses themselves, simply treating an existing infection does not guarantee that you will prevent future infections or that you will actually be able to eradicate the current infection.

When I conclude that my patient has chronic sinusitis, I will usually refer him or her to an ENT specialist, who may use an endoscope guided through the nose to check for blockage and collect samples for analysis. Not infrequently, chronic sinusitis does not resolve with traditional medical approaches, and surgery may be needed. For example, if the chronic sinusitis is due to physical changes inside the nose, antibiotics are not going to completely clear an infection. If surgical intervention is indicated, it is usually best to do it earlier rather than later. It should not be seen as the option of last resort, but as an option to prevent more extensive damage to the sinus cavities.

New, less invasive techniques have made sinus surgery safer and easier. Endoscopic sinus surgery threads a tube through the nose into the sinuses. Doctors can evaluate the sinuses' interior condition as well as clean and drain the sinuses. If needed, the same procedure can be used to remove obstructing growths or enlarge existing openings to improve drainage and breathing.

Keep in mind that even after successful surgical treatment, medical treatment to control allergies and inflammation is usually still needed.

TREATMENT PLAN: CHRONIC SINUSITIS

ANTIHISTAMINE

- Do not use traditional sedating antihistamines because they may harden mucus in sinus canals.
- Nonsedating antihistamines such as Claritin or Allegra can be used if allergies are provoking chronic sinusitis.

DECONGESTANTS

- Oral decongestant such as pseudoephrine can be used if it does not cause undue increase in blood pressure or insomnia.
- Due to chronic nature of symptoms, do not rely on spray decongestants, which can only be used for three days.

ANTI-INFLAMMATORY

- Steroid sprays such as Fluticasone can be prescribed if chronic sinusitis is due to allergies.
- If more relief is needed, new antiallergy medications such as antileukotrienes (Singulair) or mast cell inhibitors (Intal) can be prescribed.
- Acetaminophen, ibuprofen, or aspirin can be used twice a day to temporarily relieve headache.

COUGH CONTROL

- If cough is present, it is due to the drip of mucus from congested sinus passages. Rather than simply mask cough reflex, it is important to deal directly with the underlying chronic sinusitis.

Antibiotics

- Antibiotics such as Augmentin or Levaquin are prescribed for four to six weeks—far longer than the traditional five to seven days for most other upper respiratory infections.
- If problems do not seem to be getting better or symptoms return shortly after treatment ends, a different antibiotic such as a quinolone like Levaquin can be prescribed for another four to six weeks.
- If sinusitis does not respond to either antibiotic, aerosolized antifungal therapy may be necessary.

Vaccines

- None available.

Antiviral Drugs

- Not applicable.

Nutritional Therapy

- Regular meals plus:
  - chicken soup once a day.
  - two to three cups hot tea daily.
  - four to five servings of cold water, tea, diet soda, a day.

Hydrotherapy

- Nasal rinse with handheld spray or automatic irrigator twice a day.
- In dry air conditions, use room humidifier in bedroom at night.
- Hot shower in the morning.
- Ice packs if pain develops.

Supplements

- None indicated.

Prevention of Chronic Sinusitis

The best way to avoid chronic sinusitis problems is to take proper care of colds and allergies that lead to permanently obstructed airways.

When a cold does strike, make an all-out effort to handle congestion. Drink liquids to thin mucus, spray decongestants into the nose to shrink swollen airways, and use a saline nasal spray to dissolve dry, hardened mucus. If the cold lasts more than a week to ten days, call your doctor. He or she will be able to prescribe anti-inflammatory sprays, or if necessary, a short course of antibiotics.

Don't suffer for weeks before seeking medical care. This delay will make sinus problems much harder to treat effectively. The inflammation and swelling can lead to changes in the sinus bones that obstruct the already tiny drainage holes.

If you have allergies, treat them regularly and not just when you feel congested. Use allergy medication daily, not only to control symptoms, but to prevent the silent changes in the cells and airways that will lead to a full-blown sinus problem. When allergies are the trigger, as mentioned previously, I often prescribe anti-inflammatory sprays and oral medications to control the release of allergic mediators such as histamines and leukotrienes.

CHAPTER 6

Bronchitis—When a Cough Is More Than a Cough

New York is arguably the art capital of the world. There are more museums that display art, more galleries and auction houses that sell art, and more artists like my patient Kelsa Berger who work and live here than in any other city I know. At least once a year Kelsa calls me because a cold has developed into a cough that lingers for weeks and keeps her awake at night. Although thirty-five-year-old Kelsa has never smoked and has no history of asthma, she tends to develop bronchitis after a mild viral infection.

Bronchitis is an inflammation of the bronchi, the ever-branching airways of the lungs (see Illustration on page 15). Normally clear and smooth, they become obstructed with mucus and swollen with irritation during bronchitis (see Illustrations on page 95). Bronchitis is responsible for 34 million doctor's office visits a year in the United States.

There are actually three different forms of bronchitis: (1) acute viral or bacterial bronchitis, which can occur as part of a viral respiratory infection, such as a cold or flu; (2) chronic bronchitis, a progressive lung disorder caused by exposure to cigarette smoke or environmental irritation; (3) acute exacerbations of chronic bronchitis, often a bacterial bronchitis that oc-curs in the already compromised lungs of individuals with COPD (chronic obstructive pulmonary disease).

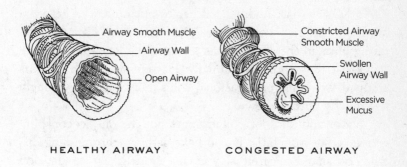

HEALTHY AIRWAY   CONGESTED AIRWAY

ACUTE VIRAL BRONCHITIS

Symptoms of Acute Viral Bronchitis

In acute bronchitis, the characteristic symptom of a cough ap-pears during a routine viral illness and lingers on, often for weeks. Studies have shown that bronchitis develops in 30 per-cent of patients with colds and 90 percent of patients with the flu. The viral infection initially irritates the surface (epithelial) lining of the airways, provoking the release of inflammatory compounds. This leads to the production of mucus and a con-striction of the airways.

Causes of Acute Bronchitis

Environmental irritation can increase your chance of develop-ing viral bronchitis. My artist patient, Kelsa, lived and worked in a large loft. She did her multimedia installations in the center of the apartment and had created a small living and sleeping area in the corner of the loft. The smell of oil paint, solvents, and welding vapors filled the entire space. When she got a viral infection, the elevated levels of these volatile pollutant chemicals triggered airway irritability and bronchitis.

In Kelsa's case, I convinced her to put up a wall between her living and her working areas, and we set up HEPA air filtering units in the studio. This lowered the level of art pollutants that Kelsa breathed in daily. Her episodes of bronchitis stopped. She still got occasional colds, but they ended simply and quietly within a few days.

Indoor and outdoor pollution are not the only coconspirators in viral bronchitis. If you have asthma, chronic lung disease, or smoke cigarettes, you are more likely to develop bronchitis with a cold or flu.

Transmission of Acute Viral Bronchitis

You don't catch bronchitis, but you can catch the cold or flu virus that produces the original infection. Using prevention techniques for these ailments, including washing your hands and getting a flu shot, will dramatically decrease your risk of developing this common viral aftermath.

Impact of Infection

The virus that causes the respiratory infection of bronchitis irritates the trachea and bronchi. The airways become congested with blood and fluid leaking from blood vessels. Increased mucus production further adds to the airway blockage. In a particularly severe viral infection, the surface of the airways may become pitted and damaged. Not infrequently, the viral-induced irritation leads to the overly sensitive airways usually seen in asthma.

Diagnosis—Everything That Coughs Is Not Bronchitis

When a patient comes in with a cough following a cold, it's important to arrive at the right diagnosis. First, I always ask about chronic nasal allergies that can cause mucus to drip down the throat and cause a cough. Asthma is also a possibility when coughing is the chief complaint. If you have a history of allergies, hay fever, or eczema, are wheezing, or have family members with asthma, I would do a pulmonary function test known as a spirometry. This simple six-second test will tell how well your lungs can take in air and blow it out rapidly. If your pulmonary function is less than expected for your age, I will measure the effect of an inhaled drug that helps asthmatic airways relax. If the improvement is small, I will suspect bronchitis, but if the relief is significant, then the diagnosis would be asthma.

Coughs can also be caused by heartburn. Excess stomach acid that is chronically refluxed into the esophagus and ultimately inhaled into the lungs will cause irritation and cough. If you tend to belch, if you wake up at night coughing, and if you tend to eat late, then it is likely that the cough is due to GERD, or gastroesophageal reflux disease. This is best treated by agents that reduce the acid level in your stomach, such as Pepcid and Prilosec.

Most patients who come to my office with a cough expect an X-ray, and they are not often disappointed. As a pulmonologist, I probably have a lower threshold for an ordinary chest X-ray because I have X-ray facilities in my office at the Mt. Sinai Faculty Practice where I see patients. However, if you're a smoker, over the age of forty, have a cough and a fever, I think that a chest X-ray is called for wherever you get medical care. Because people tend to go to doctors irregularly in these days of managed care, they are likely to have less regular health

QUICK TIP:

A cold that causes bronchitis is commonly referred to as a chest cold. Those colds whose symptoms end at the throat are called head colds.

care than in the past. An acute illness like a bronchitis can give a physician an opportunity to examine the patient and pick up a potential problem early.

If the X-ray of the chest doesn't show much, that's actually a positive sign. The absence of patchy infiltrates (white areas of increased density within the lung tissue) means it's not pneumonia and we're usually looking at a relatively superficial infection in the lungs. It will also show us any other abnormalities in the lung tissue and help us identify problems before they become serious.

It is also important to differentiate bronchitis from pleurisy. Pleurisy is an inflammation of the double-layered membranes called pleurae that line your chest cavity (see Illustration on page 15). We are totally unaware of our pleurae until they become irritated. Symptoms include chest pain with shortness of breath, a dry rather than wet cough, and sometimes chills. The chest pain becomes worse if you cough, sneeze, move, or take a deep breath. Pleurisy can occur as the result of a viral infection, a pneumonia, a blood clot, or even pancreatitis, but often the cause is unknown. Chest pain can also be a sign of more serious illness, so in some cases the doctor may need to insert a needle to remove fluid from your pleural tissues and evaluate it. If the pain is associated with a bacterial infection in the chest, such as a bacterial pneumonia, the fluid may be sterile (without bacterial growth), simply representing an irritation of the pleura by the adjacent pneumonia, or there may be an actual infection of the pleura. In the latter case, it should be treated with an appropriate antibiotic agent, adequate pain control as with acetaminophen or ibuprofen or a narcotic, and a strong cough medicine to control spasms. It may be necessary to have the bacteria-induced fluid removed with a chest tube or surgery so that the infection can clear and the pleura not be further damaged.

Preventing Viral Bronchitis

Preventing viral bronchitis starts with preventing the original cold or flu. During the cold season that runs from early fall to early spring, make sure that you wash your hands frequently. An annual flu shot will not only protect against flu, but will also lower the risk of developing debilitating bronchitis. If the flu does strike and you have a history of developing bronchitis or have underlying health problems, your doctor may prescribe antivirals such as Tamiflu or Relenza. These drugs will lessen flu symptoms, shorten illness, and possibly cease progression to bronchitis.

Treatment Issues of Viral Bronchitis

Although most cases of bronchitis are caused by a virus, or by environmental irritation, people demand and frequently get prescriptions for antibiotics. In fact 80 percent of people who come to a doctor's office with bronchitis get a prescription for antibiotics. It is estimated that 30 percent of all prescriptions written for these miracle drugs are for bronchitis, against which they probably have little effect.

The Centers for Disease Control and Prevention and the American College of Physicians have actively campaigned to discourage physicians from prescribing antibiotics for most cases of bronchitis and have launched public information campaigns to urge people not to ask for them. Health officials are concerned that overuse of antibiotics when they're not needed is leading to the development of antibiotic-resistant bacteria

TREATMENT PLAN: VIRAL BRONCHITIS

ANTIHISTAMINE

• Use traditional antihistamine as directed by manufacturer.

DECONGESTANT

• Anticholinergic nasal spray for three days, then switch to oral form of decongestant if needed.

ANTI-INFLAMMATORY

• Acetaminophen (650 mg), aspirin (500 mg), or ibuprofen (200 mg) twice a day in acute phase of illness (usually three–four days).
• Beta-agonist bronchodilator up to four times a day until cough is gone. This can be as long as six weeks.

QUELLING THE COUGH

• Over-the-counter suppressants that contain dextromethorphan or prescription formulations with codeine for three to five days. Use as directed on package.
• If cough persists for more than a week, you may need a bronchodilator such as albuterol *or* Atrovent, and anti-inflammatory sprays such as Flovent or Qvar may help.

ANTIBIOTICS

• Usually not necessary for viral bronchitis. If fever rises or mucus turns yellow or green, discuss antibiotic use with your physician.

VACCINES

- None directly for viral bronchitis. However, since up to 90 percent of people with the flu develop some degree of bronchitis, an annual flu shot will substantially cut the risk of developing post-flu bronchitis.

ANTIVIRAL DRUGS

- Antiviral medications such as Tamiflu used in the first forty-eight hours of the flu have been shown to cut the risk of developing complications such as bronchitis. They are not directly helpful for treating viral bronchitis.

NUTRITIONAL THERAPY

- Regular meals.
- If you like and can tolerate spicy foods, try tomato juice with horseradish, hot and sour soup, or hot sauce on scrambled eggs to loosen airway congestion.
- Drink three to four cups hot tea a day. Flavor with honey and lemon to soothe cough-irritated throat.

HYDROTHERAPY

- Hot showers in the morning to loosen mucus in airways.
- If congested during the day, use steam inhaler with eucalyptus extract.
- Keep well hydrated with room humidifier.
- Drink four to five glasses of fluid a day.

SUPPLEMENTS

- None indicated effective.

and that in the near future we may have no effective antibiotics when we desperately need them for true bacterial infections.

Current guidelines for healthy people encourage doctors not to routinely prescribe antibiotics for bronchitis. However, when a person has underlying health problems such as diabetes or heart disease, or is a smoker, antibiotics may be a more appropriate choice since bacterial superinfection is much more common. This is a discussion you need to have with your physician.

In my practice if I am comfortable that the diagnosis is viral bronchitis, I select the treatment of choice today, which is a bronchodilator that opens the airways and relieves the irritation in the bronchi.

ACUTE BACTERIAL BRONCHITIS

Causes and Symptoms of Acute Bacterial Bronchitis

The lower airways are normally sterile, that is to say, free of germs. Most acute bacterial bronchitis begins as a viral bronchitis. Viral infection of the airways damages the airway mucosa and make it more susceptible to bacterial invasion.

If you have chronic airway disease such as chronic bronchitis or asthma, your airways are always irritated and damaged and are more likely to develop a bacterial bronchitis with a cold or flu.

In addition to an exhausting cough, symptoms of bacterial bronchitis include a high fever several days after the low-grade fever of the original cold or flu virus has subsided. Phlegm production increases and the color changes from clear and thin to thicker and cloudy or greenish yellow. This change in color represents the result of white blood cells dying as they devour countless bacteria and leaving behind a residue of cellular debris (mostly DNA). In addition, the disease-fighting mechanisms of the body provoke the release of prostaglandins, which lead to higher fever.

In bacterial bronchitis that follows viral bronchitis or develops in damaged airways, the excess mucus in swollen, irritated airways becomes a perfect place for bacteria, such as *streptococcus* or *Staphylococcus aureus,* to grow. These bacteria are commonly present in our upper airways and are just waiting for situations such as a cold or flu to make their presence known. We don't catch bacterial bronchitis from others, but rather infect ourselves.

Diagnosis of Bacterial Bronchitis

The history of the original illness (usually a viral respiratory infection or underlying chronic bronchitis or asthma) plus the development of new symptoms such as fever suggest that the viral bronchitis (or the chronic bronchitis) has now worsened and developed into a bacterial illness. A blood test will show an elevated white count with an increase in cells called *polymorphonuclear leukocytes* (PMN), a clear sign of an infection. Examination of the sputum by Gram's stain usually shows many white blood cells and bacteria. The X-ray can have what we call a "dirty appearance." The bronchi look a bit thickened, and the small, scratchy lines called markings on the lungs increase. On any lung X-ray there are always markings. When there is inflammation, the number of markings can go up.

Preventing Bacterial Bronchitis

To prevent a bacterial bronchitis from developing after viral invasion, start by drinking plenty of hot tea and soup to thin mucus in the airways. Bacteria like to grow in thickened, older mucus, and besides, it is important to keep the body hydrated. Hot showers and steam will aid in removing dry, hardened mu-

TREATMENT PLAN: BACTERIAL BRONCHITIS

ANTIHISTAMINES

- Not necessary.

DECONGESTANTS

- Not necessary.

ANTI-INFLAMMATORY

- Use acetaminophen, ibuprofen, or aspirin two or three times a day for fever.

QUELLING THE COUGH

- Start with cough medication that contains dextromethorphan or codeine.
- If cough persists, use a bronchodilator such as Atrovent three or four times a day for up to six weeks.

ANTIBIOTICS

- Augmentin or Levaquin for five to seven days.

cus from the upper and lower airways. Doctors no longer prescribe antibiotics to *prevent* bacterial bronchitis. It doesn't seem to work and can lead to increased bacterial resistance.

Treatment of Bacterial Bronchitis

Treatment is aimed at controlling both the infection and symptoms. A broad-spectrum antibiotic, such as Augmentin or Levaquin, which are specific for the types of bacteria known to

Vaccines

- An annual flu shot will prevent the most common viral infection that leads to bacterial bronchitis.

Antiviral Drugs

- Medications such as Relenza or Tamiflu may be prescribed to limit flu symptoms to prevent development of bacterial bronchitis if you are at higher risk of developing complications.

Nutritional Therapy

- Regular meals plus:
  - one cup of hot soup a day.
  - two to three cups hot tea a day.
  - three to four cups water, juice, or diet soda, a day.
  - one serving of a spicy item such as tomato juice with horseradish, or hot and sour soup (optional).

Hydrotherapy

- Hot shower in the morning.
- If air is especially dry, portable room humidifier at night.
- Saline gargle one or two times a day to quiet cough reflex in throat.

occur in bacterial bronchitis, can be taken for five to seven days. Medications to keep airways open called bronchodilators will help you breathe easier, help cough out infected mucus, and reduce coughing by ridding the airway of irritating material.

CHRONIC BRONCHITIS

Chronic bronchitis occurs due to long-term lung damage from cigarette smoking and/or high levels of environmental pollutants. Often called smoker's cough, it affects an estimated 12 million Americans and is characterized by a cough that lingers literally for years, an increase in phlegm, and a growing shortness of breath. Chronic bronchitis is a form of lung disease known as COPD or chronic obstructive pulmonary disease.

Although chronic bronchitis is currently the fourth leading cause of death in the United States, few people in the country have ever heard of it. In most cases, people with this disease consult me for relief of an annoying cough. They are often shocked to learn that they have a progressive and chronic disease.

Causes of Chronic Bronchitis

Chronic bronchitis is a chronic, progressive lung disease that is thought to be caused by years of inflammation due to tobacco exposure. While environmental exposures such as occupational air pollution are also linked to chronic bronchitis, it is safe to say that without cigarettes, chronic bronchitis would not be the problem it is in the United States.

When the lung is repeatedly exposed to tobacco smoke, a number of changes develop. As you inhale, the mucus glands become enlarged, and new glands appear in new areas, leading to increased production of the sticky fluid. The airways become irritated by the mucus, and the irritation triggers coughing, the body's way of trying to clear the mucus. This is the well-known "smoker's cough." To make matters worse, cigarette smoke paralyzes the cilia, so that they can no longer clear the mucus out of the airways. The resulting accumulation of bacteria and pollutants creates more inflammation and infection.

It gets even worse. This inflammation in the airways trig-

SECONDHAND SMOKE

According to the Centers for Disease Control and Prevention, fifty thousand people die each year from exposure to other people's cigarettes. We know that growing up in a home where there is cigarette smoking leads to a greater risk of developing asthma and chronic bronchitis. Don't smoke around others, and don't let others light up around you.

gers the defense system, which rushes white blood cells to engulf invading bacteria and dirt particles. The presence of these cells leads the airways to become scarred, thickened, and irritable—a process we call *remodeling*. Eventually the airways become narrowed, which makes breathing more difficult—hence shortness of breath.

Transmission of Chronic Bronchitis

Keep in mind that chronic bronchitis is not an infectious disease. We believe that there is an underlying genetic tendency to develop problems in response to exposure to tobacco smoke, but we don't know who is vulnerable. The only way to avoid chronic lung disease is to stay away from smoking. If you don't smoke, don't start. If you do smoke, it is important to stop.

Diagnosis of Chronic Bronchitis

By definition, chronic bronchitis is a productive cough that lingers three months, two years in a row. An X-ray might show thickened airways and increased marking on the lungs. The person's sputum could be blood-streaked, which does not mean that the lungs are bleeding, but that small blood vessels have ruptured from extended periods of coughing.

One of the most important clues to chronic bronchitis is the

THE SIX-SECOND TEST THAT CAN SAVE YOUR LIFE

A simple, painless, inexpensive test can measure how well your lungs are working. Known as a spirometry, it can provide your doctor with information that may just save your life. Before testing, I will enter your vital statistics—age, weight, height, race, and sex. This will provide me with a set of predicted results for these characteristics. To perform this test, you blow into a mouthpiece attached to a device that measures airflow. The resulting numbers will give me a snapshot of how well your lungs function.

The American Thoracic Society recommends that a spirometry should be part of an annual physical for current and former smokers over age forty. A spirometry can pick up problems before they cause symptoms and loss of lung function.

person's smoking history. We measure exposure to cigarettes in terms of "pack years"—the number of years that you have smoked multiplied by the average number of packs smoked per day. For example, if you have been smoking for ten years and you smoke one pack a day, that is equal to ten pack years. Surveys indicate that health problems usually appear at around twenty pack years, but that does not mean you can keep smoking safely until you have reached the magic number twenty. Damage from tobacco exposure occurs during all the years that you are smoking. At around twenty pack years, clearly defined disease states develop. The earlier you stop, the more you will lower your risk of developing smoking-related health problems.

Prevention of Chronic Bronchitis

Sometimes it seems cigarette smoking is the seven-hundred-pound gorilla sitting on my desk. It's an overwhelming health issue, but a delicate subject to raise with my patients. Smoking is an important cause of chronic bronchitis, and most people recognize that quitting smoking is vital to healthy lungs. What is less well-known is the importance of diet and exercise to strong and fit airways.

For over forty years researchers have demonstrated links between diet and the risk of high blood pressure, diabetes, heart disease, and some types of cancers. Now studies suggest that diet can be important in reducing the chances of developing lung disease. Doctors have found that people whose diets were high in fruits and vegetables had lower rates of asthma and chronic lung disease—even in people who smoked.

A study of the eating habits of nine thousand Americans found that people with low blood levels of vitamin C had even higher incidence of bronchitis. A related study at Johns Hopkins University found that men and women with low vitamin A levels had higher incidence of obstructed airways. Moreover, the Third National Health and Nutrition Examination Survey (NHANESIII) found that people with a high vitamin E intake had better lung function.

Given these interesting results, the next step was to see if supplements of vitamin C, E, or A would offer the same pulmonary benefits. A joint study from the National Public Health Institute in Finland followed the health of thirty thousand men who regularly smoked cigarettes. One group was given vitamins, while another received placebos (sugar pills). At the end of the six-year study it was disappointing to find no differences in pulmonary health between the groups.

The results of the Beta-Carotene and Retinol Efficiency Study (CARET) study, which followed the health of eighteen thousand people at risk for lung cancer, were even more troubling. Participants who were given beta-carotene supplements had a *40 percent increase* in lung cancer mortality. Equally frightening, the men in the CARET study receiving supplements

showed a *30 percent increase* in mortality from all causes including heart disease.

What went wrong? Some doctors suggested that the doses
of supplements were wrong, while other experts felt that the
studies were too short to show benefits. At this point we
know that diets rich in fruits and vegetables, not vitamin supplements, provide pulmonary benefits. To lower risk of developing chronic bronchitis, try to eat five to seven servings of
nutrient-rich fruits and vegetables each day.

The Air in Here

The Environmental Protection Agency (EPA) estimates that
the air quality inside our homes and offices is on average two to
five times worse than that outdoors. On every floor and in
every room of your home there are irritants to the lungs. Our
energy-efficient homes may lower heating bills, but they tend to
seal up indoor pollutants. Dirt, animal dander and hairs, mold,
bacteria, and pollen can build to highly irritating levels.

We spend up to 90 percent of our time indoors. To keep
home air quality healthy, it is essential to improve ventilation.
In the spring and summer, run the air conditioner to remove air
pollutants and moisture from your home. A good air conditioner should even remove larger irritant particles such as
smoke and pollen. A portable air-cleaning unit with a HEPA
filter removes 95 percent of even the smallest pollutant particles. Some brands of HEPA air cleaners such as those made by
Honeywell remove over 95 percent of bacteria from the air.

Treatment Issues of Chronic Bronchitis

Chronic bronchitis is treated differently from other respiratory
illnesses. The goal is not just to relieve symptoms temporarily,
but to establish a program of care to keep airways working
smoothly. I may prescribe long-acting inhaled bronchodilators

ANOTHER OZONE LAYER
TO WORRY ABOUT

Other air cleaners offered for controlling air quality are not nearly as effective as HEPA air cleaners. Ionizing air cleaners are designed to clear the air by ionizing particles in the air and having them settle on the walls and floors. The particles are soon stirred up by activity and room currents and return to the air you are inhaling. Some models of ionizing air cleaners give off ozone, which is itself a particularly dangerous lung irritant. A study published in the Journal of Applied Occupational and Environmental Hygiene found that some models of ionizing air cleaners produce ozone at levels that exceeded EPA air quality standards.

like Spiriva that help to keep the airways open for twenty-four hours. If running for a bus or losing your wallet make you feel suddenly breathless, short-acting "rescue" bronchodilators such as Atrovent can be of help. When allergies and/or asthma are also present, I can add an inhaled steroid such as Pulmicort or a combination bronchodilator and steroid such as Advair to reduce both inflammation and bronchoconstriction. If mucus secretions are particularly bothersome, an old but effective drug called theophylline has been shown to be effective.

We are also now recognizing that exercise is important for pulmonary health. Regular physical activity builds strength and muscle, and a trained body has lower oxygen needs. As a result the lungs do not need to work as hard—a major plus for airways already stressed by chronic bronchitis.

Exercise need not be long and punishing. Scheduling thirty-minute exercise sessions three to four times a week will offer your lungs critical benefits.

TREATMENT PLAN: CHRONIC BRONCHITIS

ANTIHISTAMINE

• Not required.

DECONGESTANT

• Not required.

ANTI-INFLAMMATORY

• Inhaled steroid sprays such as Flovent and Qvar.
• Bronchodilators:
  ▪ Short-acting: albuterol, Atrovent.
  ▪ Long-acting: Serevent, Spiriva.
  ▪ Theophylline.

QUELLING THE COUGH

• Cough suppressants containing codeine.

ANTIBIOTICS

• Prescribed for respiratory infection to treat (early) acute exacerbations.

VACCINES

• Annual flu shot.
• Pneumonia vaccine every ten years.

ANTIVIRAL DRUGS

• Tamiflu or Relenza can be prescribed if flu symptoms develop (first one to two days).

NUTRITIONAL THERAPY

- Diets high in fruits and vegetables have been shown to lower the risk of chronic bronchitis.

HYDROTHERAPY

- Hot shower to humidify and loosen dry secretions.

OTHER

- Avoid secondhand smoke.
- Exercise indoors two to three times a week.
- Improve air quality in your home by removing carpets; use a HEPA air cleaner.
- If your home has a dog or cat, don't let it into your bedroom.

ACUTE EXACERBATION OF CHRONIC BRONCHITIS

When properly treated, people with chronic bronchitis can feel good most of the time. While you might not be able to win a 10K race, working, playing, and traveling can be comfortable and enjoyable. Then for reasons we don't completely understand, an acute flare-up of symptoms may occur that can lead to a medical crisis called an *acute exacerbation*. Often, such an episode is what leads you to discover you have chronic bronchitis.

Symptoms of an acute exacerbation are usually not subtle. You develop an increased shortness of breath, increase in coughing, and a troubling increase in phlegm. In some cases there is an almost desperate need for air.

Acute exacerbations often start with a minor viral illness like a cold or flu. For my patient Carla Penny, I could almost mark on my calendar when she would call me with symptoms of an acute exacerbation. Around each Christmas and Easter, Carla would call with the classic symptom of shortness of breath. In addition to being a well-known writer for women's magazines, Carla was the matriarch of her family and adored by her many grandchildren. In December and April, Carla would have a household full of her offspring's offspring.

You don't catch acute exacerbations, but you can catch the virus or bacteria that provokes it. I began to suspect that Carla's large brood of beautiful grandchildren could be a source of her holiday infections. We gave all the kids and their parents flu shots and discussed the signs and symptoms of colds and sore throats. They all recognized that a visit with Grandma would need to be postponed if there were signs of sniffles or a sore throat. It's been five years, and Carla has had only a single mild exacerbation.

Acute exacerbations can also be provoked by exposure to high levels of environmental pollution or natural allergens. Harry Learner is a bicoastal producer who tends to develop acute exacerbations in sunny California rather than rainy New York. His problems tend to correspond with high levels of ozone that occur in the heat and humidity of a Southern California summer.

For Harry, the solution was even easier—avoid L.A. when smog was a problem. He, too, has remained healthy and busy.

Impact of Infection on Chronic Bronchitis

An infection causes the mucous glands to work overtime. The walls of the airways swell and bacterial levels rise. The body responds by producing inflammatory compounds such as interleukin and bradykinin that irritate the airways, causing them to contract—thus resulting in shortness of breath. Keep in mind it's not the infection or irritation that is the problem, it is the airways' reaction to these situations.

Diagnosis of Acute Exacerbation of Chronic Bronchitis

Listening to your history of environmental exposures and your current symptoms, I suspect an acute exacerbation of chronic bronchitis. A chest X-ray is usually not dramatically changed (unless there is pneumonia), and the white blood count will be fairly normal. A test with a spirometer will give me a better idea of how well your lungs can take in and blow out air. In an acute exacerbation, I frequently see a lower-than-expected number, indicating that the lungs are having trouble exhaling through narrowed airways.

If you have waited several days before calling me, a secondary bacterial infection may have set in. Bacterial pneumonia can develop and with it symptoms of chest pain and fever. Be aware that an acute exacerbation can be a serious, even fatal illness. Hospitalization is not unusual. In some cases we need to admit patients to the intensive care unit, and even with all the support and technology available in hospitals today, a patient hospitalized with an acute exacerbation has a 10 percent risk of mortality.

Prevention of an Acute Exacerbation

In lung disease, as in football, the best defense is a good offense. Make an annual flu shot as much a part of your autumn as watching foliage change and drinking fresh apple cider. Follow the recommended CDC guidelines for vaccination in chapter 3 to see if you should get vaccinated for both influenza and pneumonia.

At the first sign of the critical trio of symptoms—increased shortness of breath, increased cough, and increased phlegm—call your physician. Don't worry about bothering us. We love to tell patients that they are not sick. What we do find frustrating is when you don't call until you need the emergency room.

If you have chronic bronchitis or are a long-term smoker, it is important to get early and thorough care. Each episode of acute exacerbation may permanently reduce your lung function. Preventing these flare-ups will keep you active and healthy.

Treatment Issues for Acute Exacerbations

If you call me at the first sign of the symptoms, I will immediately prescribe a five-to-seven-day course of broad-spectrum antibiotics. In addition, I might prescribe oral steroids, which appear to reduce airway inflammation, and which when combined with antibiotics can short-circuit the exacerbation. If you don't respond within a day or two and still feel breathless, I might admit you to the hospital to be able to provide oxygen, antibiotics, bronchodilators, and anti-inflammatory steroids given intravenously.

CHAPTER 7

STREP THROAT—WHEN IT EVEN HURTS TO SWALLOW

M y neighbor Gordon Duff loved being Emily's father. When she was born, he cherished the quiet of 3 a.m. feedings. He loved the excuse that fatherhood gave him to get down on the floor and play with action figures. On Sundays, he now had a loyal companion who would sit with him and watch football. But when Emily went off to preschool, Gordon discovered something painful about parenting. One evening he came to my door. Holding his throat with one hand and gesturing wildly with the other, he pleaded for "anything to end this mother of all sore throats."

Sore throats are the sixth leading cause of doctor's office visits in the United States. There are 18 million cases a year, but only 10 to 20 percent of these sore throats are strep throat, yet at least 75 percent of people who consult a doctor for a sore throat receive antibiotics.

Sore throat is a subjective term that refers to pain in the back of the mouth, and pain on swallowing. Frequently it accompanies an upper respiratory viral infection, such as influenza or colds, or even develops when there is a great deal of coughing, such as during pneumonia or bronchitis.

Some sore throats are caused by viruses, and others, unaccompanied by symptoms of congestion, are caused by bacteria. The most feared, and probably the most painful, type of sore throat is caused by different forms of streptococcus bacteria and is commonly known as strep throat.

The peak season for strep throat is in the early spring. The main concerns about strep throat, in addition to its discomfort, are the serious complications. It can lead to a heart disease known as *rheumatic fever*, or a kidney disorder called *glomerulonephritis*. These diseases are much less common than they used to be, yet we still have a historical fear that these serious and life-threatening complications will develop. Today, however, doctors are more concerned about the overuse of antibiotics in treating strep throat, not only because they are expensive, but because of the increasing problem of bacterial resistance.

When antibiotics were first introduced in the 1940s, infections that were often fatal became minor, short-lived problems. For a short time, doctors thought that bacterial illness had been eliminated. They were wrong. Within a decade, bacteria began developing ways to thrive in spite of the presence of an antibiotic.

Resistance can take different forms. For example, some resistant bacteria produce chemicals that inactivate antibiotics, while others actually pump antibiotics out of infected cells before they can take effect. Even more troubling, resistance strategies to antibiotics can be shared among bacteria as genetic material from resistant bacteria is transferred to other still vulnerable organisms.

Stopping the development and spread of resistant bacteria has become a critical goal for the medical community. Because the more antibiotics are used, the more resistance will develop, national health organizations have developed guidelines to curb unnecessary use of antibiotics. Survey research indicates the upper respiratory infections such as sore throat are frequently treated with unnecessary antibiotics.

When I treat patients with a sore throat, I have to weigh relief of their symptoms against the risks of their developing resistant bacteria. I want to ensure that if a serious bacterial illness does develop in the future, they will still be sensitive to the antibiotics that I will use to cure them.

Causes of Strep Throat

The streptococcus bacteria were first discovered in the 1880s. The name (from the Greek *strep* for "chain" and *coccus* for "round") describes how these chubby balls grow in pearl-like chains or pairs. There are literally hundreds of types of streptococci, which cause a wide range of problems including impetigo, rheumatic fever, and kidney disease. In fact, over eighty different types of strep can cause pneumonia.

Three types of strep can cause sore throats, but only the Group A streptococcus is of such concern that doctors feel it should be treated with antibiotics. Groups C and G do not cause complications of rheumatic fever or glomerulonephritis. To control development of resistant antibiotics, these should not be treated aggressively, but just for symptomatic relief.

Symptoms of a Strep Throat

To make the diagnosis of a strep throat, the American College of Physicians has developed four key signs and advises that at least three of these should be present. I agree with the guidelines and I look for:

- Painful throat
- Swollen glands on either side of the throat or under the chin
- Redness of the throat
- White patches and swelling on the tonsils

Headache, chills, and stomach pain are also common symptoms. In a strep throat, cough and congestion are usually absent. If these symptoms are prominent, it suggests to me that the problem is a virus rather than streptococcus.

A Ruthless Enemy

Doctors rate the strength of bacteria on three factors: how well they can adhere to our cells; how well they can evade our natural defense systems; and how much tissue damage they cause. Given how miserable you can feel with a strep throat, it's not surprising that in these three "enemy" factors, the streptococcus rates high.

Strep contains sticky proteins that easily attach to a cell matrix—the glue that holds cells together. Once attached, they secrete a protein that camouflages them from our immune system.

White blood cells, which are our first line of defense against infection, act by catching and gobbling up invading organisms. Streptococci bacteria are covered with a slimy coating that allows them to slip by the protective white blood cells—sort of like a "greased pig" defense.

Strep also release a number of enzymes, all bad: *streptokinase* causes inflammation that breaks down tissue; *streptolysin* allows the bacteria to punch holes in cells to create local inflammation; DNase breaks down our essential DNA protein, further clogging congested areas. White blood cells rush to clean up the cellular debris, leading to more inflammation, pus formation on tonsils, and high fever.

Diagnosis of Strep Throat

Unlike the cold or flu, where we make what is called an empirical diagnosis based on the clinical symptoms, a suspicion of strep throat calls for additional information. There are two fairly quick and effective tests. One is the classic "throat culture," in which the clinician takes a sample of fluid from the back of the throat with a cotton swab, inserts the swab in a carrier tube, and sends it to a lab for analysis. The answer will come back in forty-eight hours.

The throat culture was developed in 1954. Most physicians of that era, such as my father, used to do throat cultures in their office. My father was a physician who escaped from Nazi-occupied Paris and set up a general practice in the South Bronx in New York City. We lived in the back of his office on Avenue Saint John. Before he went to sleep at night, he would often check on the status of the throat cultures in his tiny office incubator. If I heard him walk down the short hall to his office, I would get out of bed and follow him to the incubator. He would show me the petri dishes and I would try to identify the different organisms.

The Clinical Laboratories Improvement Act of 1988 deterred physicians from their convenient albeit modest office-based labs. In the 1980s the Centers for Disease Control estimated that up to 36 million throat cultures were performed annually. Since that high point the numbers of throat cultures have dropped significantly as other diagnostic methods have become more popular.

A newer test is the RAT, or rapid antigen test, which allows me to test for the streptococcus antigen in my office and have the answer in twenty minutes. To perform the test I take a swab sample from your throat and insert it in a tube with a solution that will register if you have formed antibodies to fight streptococcus A.

The RAT is considered somewhat less reliable than the throat culture, with a greater incidence of false negatives. In other words, it can indicate that strep are not a problem when they are actually causing an infection. Still, because it is quicker and less expensive, doctors generally start with a RAT. If it is positive, they know that they are dealing with Group A strep and will treat accordingly. If it is negative, they will then proceed with a throat culture.

The American Heart Association, the American Academy

GARGLE AWAY THROAT PAIN

Rinsing the throat with a mild salt solution dissolves strep-laden mucus in the throat. It provides immediate relief as it slows down the infection. Add one-quarter teaspoon kosher salt to one-half cup warm water. Tilt your head back, gargle for the count of five, then spit out all the salty water.

of Pediatrics, and the Infectious Disease Society of America all advocate that the throat culture remain the gold standard for the diagnosis of strep. Although it takes one or two days to get back the results, the delay should not cause increased risk of rheumatic disease, since at least nine days elapse between onset and the time of risk of cardiac or kidney complications. If you are uncomfortable, I may prescribe antibiotic therapy immediately, while I wait for culture results, especially if all four signs of strep are present.

Transmission of Strep Throat

Strep is an airborne bacteria spread by droplets from infected people in crowded conditions. In addition, this tenacious bacteria can be spread by hand-to-hand contact. In schools and in military camps, strep is a frequent problem. Children have a greater susceptibility to strep. Like Gordon, most adults who develop strep infections do so because of their exposure to their children. Others, such as teachers and child care workers, are exposed on the job.

Outbreaks of strep throat in community settings such as colleges or other institutions have also been linked to strep contamination in the food. The symptoms are not gastrointestinal as is usual with contaminated food, but will produce standard symptoms of fever and sore throat. If there seem to be frequent outbreaks of strep throat in your community, or if your family gets repeated cases, there may be a carrier in the community or your home. In some situations, a family member who had either an untreated or undertreated strep infection no longer experiences symptoms but can spread illness to others.

There is some debate about how long one remains infectious with or without antibiotic treatment. One of the reasons given for antibiotic treatment of strep throat is that it reduces transmission to other members of the family and in the community. Shedding of the bacteria declines quickly in adults, but can continue for much longer in children. Some people may be carriers of strep without having active symptoms, but may transmit it almost indefinitely to other people. Some doctors suggest this is what causes continual outbreaks of strep in a day care center, school, hospital, or military base.

Prevention of Strep Throat

Because it is a bacteria, strep is susceptible to antibacterial cleansers. Thorough hand washing is thought to reduce the spread of strep in a community. In addition, some pediatricians recommend that the entire family be given antibiotics to protect them against developing strep when there is an outbreak in the home.

Treatment Issues of Strep Throat

The gold standard for treating strep is the antibiotic penicillin. It can be given as a single shot or as a ten-day course of oral drugs. If a patient is allergic to penicillin, other antibiotics such as erythromycin are effective. If a sore throat persists more than a week after antibiotic treatment, it is important to have additional testing. A severe sore throat that doesn't go away could be a sign of Epstein-Barr virus or mononucleosis, more serious diseases that need different care.

TREATMENT PLAN: STREP THROAT/TONSILLITIS

ANTIHISTAMINE

- Not required.

DECONGESTANT

- Not required.

ANTI-INFLAMMATORY

- Acetaminophen, ibuprofen, or aspirin two or three times a day.
- Throat lozenges or spray containing benzocaine (or other topical anesthetic) to temporarily numb sore throat pain.

QUELLING THE COUGH

- Cough not part of a strep throat.

ANTIBIOTICS

- Ten-day course of penicillin.
- Biaxin or Zithromax if there is allergy to penicillin.

Strep sore throats last about a week. The fever disappears within seven days, and the pain disappears shortly after that. However, it may take several weeks for the tonsils and the glands to return to normal. Glands and tonsils that continue to be enlarged create an uncomfortable sensation of fullness. Swallowing, while not difficult, can still feel different for a time after the infection is gone.

Vaccine

- None available.

Antiviral Drugs

- None available.

Nutritional Therapy

- Light meals at first, then regular diet.
- One serving hot chicken soup a day.
- Two to three glasses iced tea and cold water daily.
- Two to three cups hot tea with honey and lemon daily.
- Avoid spicy foods, which irritate the throat.

Hydrotherapy

- Saline gargle twice a day.
- Room humidifier in bedroom if air is cold and dry.

Supplements

- None indicated.

Complications of Strep Throat

A strep throat can lead to a serious heart disease known as *rheumatic fever*. One to five weeks after the original infection starts, the aggressive bacteria causes widespread inflammation. There is a cross-reaction between the bacterial cell walls and the patient's own tissues. It can cause pain and swelling in the joints, hence the name rheumatic fever. Often rheumatic fever affects the muscle of the heart called the myocardium. This can lead to heart failure with symptoms of shortness of breath and swelling of the legs. Rheumatic fever can affect the valves of the heart, which can become permanently scarred as they heal. As a result the heart swells and works less efficiently. Even more troubling, susceptible individuals can get rheumatic fever again and again. Each time there can be more damage to the heart and joints, until the heart is unable to function.

When I was in medical school at Bellevue, rheumatic fever was far more common than it is today. The hospital had a rheumatic fever clinic, where children who had recovered from the infection would come every two weeks for a shot of long-acting penicillin to prevent another strep infection. They would need to take the antibiotic until they were around twenty, when a more mature immune system would make them less susceptible to additional attacks.

Rheumatic fever has been on the decline in most parts of the world, but it still occurs, even in countries with the best medical care. There has been an even greater decline of a deadly kidney disease that can follow strep throat. Called *glomerulonephritis,* it is thought to be an immune response to the strep bacteria. The immune system attacks the bacteria with antibodies, but these combine with the bacteria in such a way as to form large molecular complexes that clog up the glomeruli, the filtering channels in the kidneys. Debris builds up, preventing normal function. Symptoms include swelling of the face, arms, and legs, bloody urine, and a rise in blood pressure. In many cases, dialysis is needed to support the patient until the disease can be brought under control. Fortunately, treatment with antibiotics within seven to nine days of the start of a strep infection can completely prevent the arrival of these two former childhood killers.

CHAPTER 8

PNEUMONIA—WHEN A COLD
TURNS SERIOUS

Tom Miller sat in my office trying to talk between bouts of coughing. The quiet, thirty-year-old computer consultant had been healthy until a cough and fever began two weeks ago. "I have tried everything except acupuncture," he whispered hoarsely. "Do you think it will help this awful cold? All this coughing is making my chest hurt, and last night I was shaking with chills."

As a pulmonologist, I have many patients who have coughs, but chest pain is a much less frequent symptom. Its presence, along with fever, is a red flag for pneumonia. "Before we discuss treatment, I would like to listen to your chest and do a chest X-ray," I answered.

Tom took off his shirt and I placed the stethoscope on his chest. As he inhaled, I could hear crackles, or rales, another key indicator of pneumonia. As I suspected, the X-ray showed a patchy infiltrate in the lower third of his right lung with shadows in the normally black spaces occupied by the air-filled lung. Tom had mycoplasma pneumonia, one of the more than thirty different types of this common but potentially serious disease.

Pneumonia affects 4 million people annually in the United States and carries a $20 billion health-care price tag. Seventy-seven thousand people die each year from pneumonia, and it is frequently preventable by a simple vaccine. Pneumonia is so serious that more than 1 million people each year are hospitalized. In spite of our ability to treat this disease with antibiotics and other treatments, it remains the sixth leading cause of death in the United States, together with influenza.

Pneumonia is defined as an infection of the lower respiratory tract. Unlike the common cold, which affects the upper airways, this infection is localized to structures deep inside the lungs. Pneumonia is a disease primarily of the smaller airways, the smaller bronchi (bronchioles) and the alveoli, the small pouches that protrude from the walls of the small bronchi where oxygen enters the blood and carbon dioxide is removed.

With more than thirty different types of pneumonia, doctors categorize the disease into two broad groups. *Community-acquired pneumonia* is exactly what it sounds like. It is a pneumonia that people acquire while living and working in their home and neighborhood. Pneumonias that develop after seventy-two hours of being in the hospital are classified as hospital-acquired or *nosocomial*.

The reason for distinguishing between these two types of infections is that the organisms involved can vary greatly. Nosocomial pneumonias tend to be caused by much more seri-

LOBAR VERSUS BRONCHIAL PNEUMONIA

Lobar pneumonia affects an entire lobe of the lung. On an X-ray this severe pneumonia appears as a completely white lobe. By contrast, bronchial pneumonia is midway between a bad bronchitis and a mild pneumonia. On an X-ray, there is a haziness around the bronchi, but pain and/or shortness of breath are usually absent.

ous types of bacteria. These are frequently gram-negative bacteria (the red-staining germs on Gram's stain such as E. coli, or pseudomonas strains). They are much more difficult to treat with antibiotics. They require special antibiotics that may have serious side effects. Moreover, they occur in people who are already sufficiently ill to be hospitalized and thus less able to fight the infection. As a result, nosocomial infections, by and large, tend to be more serious. That is not to imply that community-acquired pneumonia is something to ignore. In fact, several types of infections occur in the community that are equally or more serious than those acquired in the hospital. For example, elderly patients, particularly those living in nursing homes (which are considered communities rather than hospitals), can develop especially serious pneumonias. Because these are frail individuals with diminished natural defenses, the pneumonia can carry especially severe symptoms.

Commonly, three different types of organisms can cause pneumonia both in the community and in hospitals—bacteria, viruses, and mycoplasma.

BACTERIAL PNEUMONIA

More than 50 percent of bacterial pneumonias are caused by a bacterium called Streptococcus pneumoniae. More than a hundred different forms of Streptococcus pneumoniae and organisms of this type are frequently present in the throats of healthy people. When body defenses are down, due to age, impaired immunity, or poor health, these bacteria can multiply and damage lungs. Even in a healthy individual, extreme stress such as the loss of a job or loved one or a severe flu can weaken resistance enough to lead to the development of bacterial pneumonia.

The signs and symptoms of bacterial pneumonia are usually dramatic. Patients develop shaking, chills, chattering teeth, sweating, severe chest pain, and a cough with greenish or rusty mucus. Both heart rate and breathing become rapid. With bacterial pneumonia you look and feel acutely ill.

A far less common but more serious pneumonia is caused by *Legionella pneumophila*. Called Legionnaires' disease, it was named after an outbreak of often fatal pneumonia that broke out at an American Legion convention in Philadelphia in 1976. Occasional outbreaks still occur and are usually linked to bacteria that have grown in stagnant water in air-conditioning and ventilation systems. Legionnaires' disease appears to affect people over the age of fifty, especially if there is a history of alcohol use, cigarette smoking, or underlying heart or lung disease.

At the other end of the age spectrum, the *Haemophilus influenzae* bacterium (it's a bacterium, despite its name) causes severe respiratory illness in children under six. Symptoms start with coldlike sneezing and congestion. Within a short period, pneumonia symptoms, including cough, fever, and shortness of breath develop. It is all too common for fluid to develop in the pleural space, leading to increased pain and respiratory problems.

Symptoms of Bacterial Pneumonia

The key symptoms of bacterial pneumonia that help differentiate it from other respiratory infections are rapid onset of coughing fits, high fever, chest pain, and shortness of breath. To understand the impact of pneumonia on the body, it's helpful to understand what generates these symptoms.

First, nerves in the airways respond to irritation and inflammation with a well-known reflex we call the cough. The purpose of the cough, as we best understand it, is to move mucus and infected material from the lower respiratory tract into the upper respiratory tract and from there into the throat, where it can be swallowed or spit out. With pneumonia, a great deal of fluid and mucus accumulates in the lower airways, and the body is almost frantic to cleanse the lungs of the fluid that is obstructing their function. The coughing can become so violent that small blood vessels rupture, giving a reddish or rusty hue to the sputum.

Second, pain is an equally significant symptom of bacterial pneumonia. The lungs themselves have no pain fibers, but pain can develop from one of several causes with pneumonia. The most common cause is that coughing puts tremendous stress on the chest wall. This structure is a composite of muscles, bones, joints, and tendons that allow the chest to move in an organized fashion. When a cough occurs, there is a dramatic release of energy. The chest moves quickly, and all of these structures are compressed and can develop the equivalent of a bruise, which causes lingering pain.

Chest pain can also develop when the pneumonia infection extends to the surface of the lung, which is coated by a membrane known as the pleura. This membrane assures the smooth motion of the lungs within the chest cavity when you breathe. However, when the infection extends to the pleural space (between the lung and the chest wall), fluid can accumulate. In bacterial pneumonia, this fluid is infected with bacteria and loaded with inflammatory compounds released by white blood cells. As a result, the pleura, which has exquisitely sensitive nerve endings, becomes painful. The characteristic symptom of infection of the pleura, which is known as *pleurisy,* is severe pain when you take a deep breath or cough. The sensation is so intense that doctors may need to prescribe narcotics to provide relief.

Third, shortness of breath has many causes in pneumonia. The lungs serve as the body's source of oxygen. Twenty-one percent of the air that we breathe naturally contains oxygen. As we inhale, part of that oxygen is transferred to the blood through the alveoli, the tiny sacs that line the ends of the smaller airways. If these airways become clogged and infected with fluid and bacteria, as is the case with pneumonia, then the amount of the oxygen supplied to the body drops sharply. In

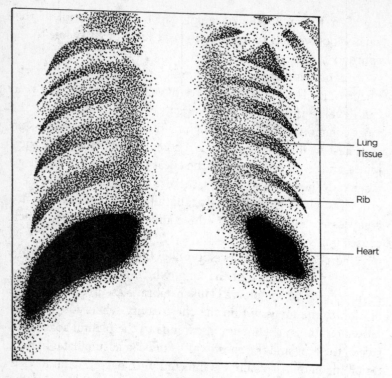

Lung
Tissue

Rib

Heart

NORMAL X-RAY

other words, the oxygen is not able to enter the necessary parts of the lung to get into the bloodstream.

With pneumonia, the lungs are working like a sponge to sop up the excess fluid. This fluid stiffens the lung, creating what we call a "restrictive pattern" in breathing. It becomes more difficult for the chest wall to move as the patient inhales, increasing the sense of shortness of breath.

Impact of the Infection

The infection in the lungs produces inflammation that causes the tissues to leak fluid from blood vessels. This fluid enters

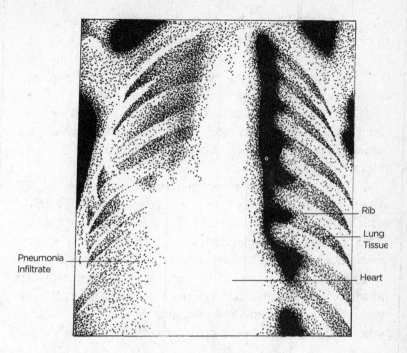

Rib

Lung
Tissue

Pneumonia
Infiltrate

Heart

BACTERIAL PNEUMONIA

what is called the interstitium of the lung. This is important tissue because, along with the alveoli, this is where oxygen enters the bloodstream. As a result, people who develop pneumonia frequently develop low oxygen content of the blood. If the pneumonia is widespread, that is, if it is in several lobes, then in addition to developing problems with oxygen, you can develop difficulties with elimination of carbon dioxide from the blood. This serious situation frequently requires oxygen supplementation. If you need just a bit of additional help, we will provide oxygen via a mask that fits over the nose and mouth. If the illness has made you too exhausted to breathe on your own, we can insert a tube into your windpipe to deliver high doses of oxygen directly into the cells.

Bacterial pneumonia is an intense battle between the bacteria and the body. The body's defenses include white blood cells and various compounds such as antibodies that help immobilize and render bacteria ineffectual, eventually killing them. As a result of these cells and compounds accumulating, the lungs may continue to look on X-ray as though the pneumonia is still on-going, even though the actual infection has cleared up. Although the patient may feel better, and the breathing is somewhat improved, the X-rays still look abnormal for weeks following pneumonia.

It is important to follow bacterial pneumonia until the X-rays completely resolve. In some people, especially those with heart or pulmonary disease, other problems may be hidden by the pneumonia and may not become apparent until the pneumonia clears up. For example, smokers who develop pneumonia may actually have a tumor in the airways that was actually part of the reason pneumonia developed in the first place. It's important to treat patients not just until they feel better, but to make sure that their chest x-ray has returned to normal.

Diagnosis of Bacterial Pneumonia

The diagnosis of bacterial pneumonia is made on the basis of patient history, X-rays, and lab tests. Because bacterial pneumonia is an infection of the lower respiratory tract, it may cause fluid to accumulate in the alveoli. Areas thus affected appear white on the X-ray (see Illustration on page 133). These are distinctive and can readily be diagnosed as pneumonia, even by a first-year medical student. In bacterial pneumonia, the shadows tend to be localized in one area, such as a lobe or segment of the lung often so well-defined that you can actually draw a pencil line around the contour of the pneumonia.

While the actual diagnosis of bacterial pneumonia is fairly straightforward, we need to characterize what kind of infection it is and what kind of bacteria are present. The first step is usually to obtain a mucus sample, one expectorated or spit out. This is more difficult than it would seem because the specimens are often mixed with a mixture of saliva and bronchial secretions, which are not representative of the infected materials from the pneumonia. It is easy to get misleading information. Once a good specimen, defined as phlegm from inside the lungs, is obtained, we can do two important tests.

First, we can make a smear, which is simply what it sounds like. We take a small amount of the expectorated mucus, spread it on a glass slide, and stain it with certain dyes that will allow us to distinguish various types of bacteria. In particular, we look to see if we are dealing with gram-positive or gram-negative bacteria. The gram-positive look blue under the microscope, and the gram-negative look red. Gram-positive and gram-negative bacteria don't just stain different colors, they also give us clues about what type of organism we are dealing with, and what type of treatment is required. The smear also allows us to confirm whether a pneumonia is caused by bacteria or some other organism.

Second, we can culture the mucus. To do this, some of the expectorated mucus is spread on a petri dish with a special growing medium. Over twenty-four to forty-eight hours, the culture will grow the kind of bacteria that are causing the infection. Most doctors, if they feel that a culture is necessary, don't like to wait until the culture results come back; they often start antibiotic treatment immediately. Still it is useful, even forty-eight hours later, to know what specific bacteria we are dealing with, and if we need to change our treatment plan.

Blood culture is another test that can be helpful, especially when patients have a high fever. Blood samples are put into culture tubes to see if the bacteria have spilled into the bloodstream. Normally the bloodstream is sterile even with an infection, so when we find bacteria in the blood, we know for certain that this is the infecting organism.

ROUND UP THE USUAL SUSPECTS

Approximately 50 percent of bacterial pneumonias are caused by *Streptococcus pneumoniae*. Other well-known bacterial culprits include *Streptococcus pyogenes,* which also causes rheumatic fever and impetigo; *Haemophilus influenzae,* which is found in the airways of most healthy adults; klebsiella, which usually causes urinary infections; pseudomonas, which tends to affect hospitalized patients; and chlamydia, which may also increase blockage in the arteries of the heart.

When an Easy Diagnosis Becomes Difficult

While the diagnosis of pneumonia is usually straightforward based on the history and a chest X-ray, sometimes confusion can occur and diagnosis be delayed. A number of conditions, particularly for "at risk" patients, such as the elderly, the very young (under age two), and people with underlying diseases, have symptoms that can mimic pneumonia's. For example, patients with heart failure can develop shadows on their X-rays, difficulty with breathing, cough, and chest pain. People who have blood clots in their lungs can develop shadows on X-rays that look exactly like pneumonia and give clinical symptoms that are closely related. In these situations, additional tests are necessary to distinguish these serious illnesses from simple pneumonia.

In patients with early-stage pneumonia, the chest X-ray may not yet show an abnormality, and this can lead the physician to draw the wrong conclusions. In patients with pneumonia who are also dehydrated, the X-ray can look normal because the fluid that normally pours into the lung tissue as a result of the infection is not available to the dehydrated body.

In congestive heart failure, the heart is not working properly and the lungs become filled with fluid, and the chest X-ray can look like that of pneumonia. In other words, fluid accumulates in the alveoli and the patient becomes short of breath and may even spit out frothy fluid. This is not sputum, but pulmonary edema fluid. However, these patients rarely have fever, complain of chest pain, or have cloudy, thickened sputum. They usually have a history of previous heart disease or actually are hospitalized due to a heart attack. The X-ray findings will tend to be much more diffuse in congestive heart failure, and the pulmonary edema will affect all parts of the lung. In contrast, bacterial pneumonia usually only affects a defined part of the lung, such as a lobe.

In the case of pulmonary embolism, where a clot lands in a blood vessel of the lung, symptoms include shortness of breath, chest pain, bloody sputum, and even a low-grade fever. While the clot itself does not cause a shadow on the chest X-ray, the bleeding associated with the clot can resemble a pneumonia. In this situation, it is essential to know what the patient has done in the days or hours before seeking medical care. Has the patient been on a long trip that required sitting in a stationary position, or has an injury kept the person in bed or fairly immobile? These situations can cause blood clots to form in the deep veins of the legs. If these clots break off a piece, that piece can be carried through the bloodstream and will usually arrive in the blood vessels of the lung, where it blocks the flow of blood through the lungs. It is also important to learn if the patient has a history of venous disease or has had a pulmonary embolism in the past.

It is also frequently difficult to diagnose pneumonia in a patient who has emphysema. Such patients have limited alveolar space, so when the infection occurs in the small airways, there is nowhere for the fluid to go. A patient with emphysema who develops pneumonia will have shortness of breath and exhaustion, but the X-ray will sometimes be unchanged because there isn't enough lung tissue in which the infected fluid can accumulate. Pneumonia can progress undiagnosed until the lungs fail and the person can no longer breathe on his or her own.

Bacterial pneumonia and acute bronchitis share a number of symptoms. Fever, cough, phlegm, and even chest pain are found with both infections. However, the X-rays are clearly different in these two respiratory infections. In bronchitis, X-rays are fundamentally normal, because the disease occurs in the bronchi, not the alveoli. In bacterial pneumonia, fluid accumulations are visible in the alveoli, clearly marking distinct areas of infection.

Serious Treatment for a Serious Disease

According to the American Thoracic Society (ATS), 75 percent of people with pneumonia can safely and effectively be treated at home. To identify when hospitalization is needed, the ATS has developed a profile of key signs that suggest direct medical care is needed.

At the top of the list is mental status. This is not an IQ test, but a measure of whether a patient can understand how to manage the pneumonia at home. When I was a first-year resident at Bellevue, I hospitalized seventy-five-year-old Edna Poole for what looked like a fairly mild pneumonia. The chief resident was furious, pointing out that her fever was barely over 101 and she didn't even need oxygen. He wanted to discharge her immediately, but I insisted that we both examine her. He just rolled his eyes, so to sweeten the deal I proposed that if he was right, I would send her home and buy him dinner at Mugs, the nearby steak house. If I was right, Edna would stay in the hospital and the dinner was on him.

When we walked into her hospital room, she was sitting up nibbling on her lunch. I waited until she had finished eating, then moved the tray away to examine her. As I put the stethoscope to her chest, she raised her head and remarked, "I smell food. They will be serving lunch soon." When I gently explained that she had just eaten lunch, she wasn't upset. "Did I enjoy it?" she asked cheerfully.

Edna stayed in the hospital for a week, and that night I had one of the best roast beef dinners I had ever eaten.

In addition to mental status, ATS guidelines suggest (either singly or in combination) that a pulse rate over 125 beats per minute (normal is 60–100), respiration rate over 20 (normal is 12–18), underlying health problems such as diabetes, and fever over 40°C (104°F) are signals that hospitalization is necessary.

One criteria for hospital care is so important that it actually stands alone. We measure the saturation of hemoglobin in the blood with oxygen (normally hemoglobin is at least 95 percent saturated with oxygen; when the level falls below 90 percent, this puts a strain on the heart and deprives tissues of needed oxygen). We use a machine called the pulse oximeter to measure this saturation. The "probe" is like a glove and slips around a finger, shining a light through the skin. This device is hooked up to a monitor that continuously displays the oxygen saturation level.

The reading gives the percentage of maximal oxygen levels. Anything from 95 to 100 percent is considered safe. Readings of 91 to 94 percent are a sign for concern. A reading of less than 90 percent or less is a sign that this pneumonia probably needs hospital care.

Once that decision is made, doctors have to judge if the patient needs to be admitted to the intensive care unit (ICU). This judgment is usually based on the patient's need for the sophisticated respiratory support that is provided in intensive care. It may be difficult to make the right decision, and patients can deteriorate rapidly with pneumonia. Despite all the technology, antibiotics, and advances in medicine, mortality for hospitalized elderly patients with pneumonia is still 20 to 25 percent.

Keep in mind that it takes a while to recover from pneumonia. Pneumonia is a serious illness, not just another respiratory infection. It requires the body to work hard to clean out debris before it can work efficiently again. As mentioned previously, the signs and symptoms of the pneumonia tend to disappear as the infection resolves, but it takes longer for the pneumonia to disappear on the actual X-ray.

Some psychological problems can occur with any major illness, and this certainly includes pneumonia. This frightening disease forces us to come to grips with our fragility and mortality. It can take weeks or even months to resolve a lingering fatigue and depression. So while the actual infection can be brought under control with a week or ten days of treatment, the consequences of pneumonia can linger for months or even longer.

One way to help your body recover from pneumonia is to make important changes in your lifestyle. We know that people who smoke and/or drink alcohol are not only more susceptible to pneumonia but also apt to have more severe forms of it. Not only do these people get more pneumonias than the average individual, but they also more frequently develop complications.

For example, one of our most fundamental airway defense mechanisms is called the muccociliary system. This is a physical barrier in the lining of the upper airways that equips the body to protect itself against inhaled viruses, dirt particles, and bacteria. All along the mucosal surface are millions of tiny hairs called cilia that beat in unison 24/7. Their synchronized motion moves material up to the mouth, into the throat where it can be spit out or swallowed. When you smoke tobacco, this mechanism is impaired. The cilia beat in chaotic motion, and the mucus that is formed is abnormal, resulting in what is called smoker's cough. Abnormal mucus doesn't have the protective effect that normal mucus does, and this makes you more susceptible to infections.

Smoking also impairs the body's immunological defenses. The white blood cells that normally exist in the lungs and the alveolar macrophages that destroy invading organisms work much less efficiently in the presence of smoke. The same holds true for alcohol. In addition to impairing body defense mechanisms, it impairs swallowing. People under the influence of alcohol commonly aspirate small amounts of food into their lungs, which can be the focus for developing a pneumonia.

Complications of Bacterial Pneumonia

When you're young and healthy, pneumonia is usually a self-limiting disease, particularly when appropriately treated in a timely manner. However, some serious complications of bacterial pneumonia should be borne in mind because they can transform a treatable disease into one with serious and long-term consequences.

Bacterial pneumonia is usually localized and affects primarily lung tissue. However, when the infection extends to the surface covering of the lung, one of two things happens. Either an inflammation occurs within the pleural space and develops into what is known as *parapneumonic effusion,* or the bacteria themselves infect this space, a problem known since the time of Hippocrates, called *empyema.*

Parapneumonic effusion may cause symptoms of pain and prolonged fever. It usually resolves without intervention, as long as the bacterial pneumonia itself is treated. However, direct infection of the pleural space constitutes a more serious complication and is essentially an abscess or boil within that area. White blood cells accumulate there, making healing much more difficult. Frequently an empyema leads to fluid buildup within this space that needs to be removed by inserting a chest tube. In severe cases surgery is necessary, to clean the pleural space of the infection.

The infection can also spread through the bloodstream. Because the lung is so rich in blood vessels, the bacteria can migrate to the bloodstream, an invasion called *bacteremia,* and infect all areas of the body. When other parts of the body become infected, it is known as *septicemia.* If the infection that began as pneumonia is transmitted to the central nervous system, it can cause meningitis or brain abscess. If it lands on the heart valves, it can cause bacterial endocarditis. All of these are serious and life-threatening and require treatment far in excess of that required for a simple bacterial pneumonia.

Preventing Bacterial Pneumonia

There is good news for prevention of bacterial pneumonia. The most common bacterial pneumonia, caused by *Streptococcus pneumoniae,* can be prevented in most cases by a simple vaccine that is usually administered once in a lifetime. This vaccine is directed against the coating of the pneumococcal organism. This coating makes it resistant to the onslaught of our white blood cells, which is why the bacteria become so virulent. The vaccine provides long-lasting protection against more than twenty-three different strains of streptococcus and is estimated to be up to 70 percent effective in people who receive it. It is recommended to all people over the age of sixty-five, and all others over the age of two with a chronic health problem such as lung or heart conditions, diabetes, or a weakened immune system, including those with HIV or undergoing treatment with steroids, chemo, or radiation. The vaccination rarely causes problems, other than maybe a little redness at the site of injection or sometimes a low fever.

The bad news is that less than 50 percent of those over age 65 who meet the recommendations for this vaccine are actually receiving it. This is one of the big holes in our communal de-

---

QUICK TIP:

Those who get the pneumonia vaccination before age sixty-five are frequently advised to get a second dose some ten years later to provide lifetime protection.

TREATMENT PLAN: BACTERIAL PNEUMONIA

ANTIHISTAMINE

• Usually not prescribed.

DECONGESTANT

• Usually not prescribed.

ANTI-INFLAMMATORY

• Acetaminophen, aspirin, or ibuprofen are prescribed to reduce fever and chest pain. If discomfort is severe, codeine or other narcotics may be ordered.

QUELLING THE COUGH

• Codeine may be prescribed if not already ordered to reduce chest pain.
• Acetylcysteine may be prescribed to thin the thickend, bacteria-laden mucus, so that the lungs can begin to heal.

ANTIBIOTICS

• Antibiotics are always necessary in bacterial pneumonia. Used for seven to ten days, top choices are Levaquin, Augmentin, Rocephin (if hospitalized), and Ceftin.

fense against pneumonia and its complications. If you only follow one piece of advice from this book, it should be to get a pneumonia vaccination if you are included in the recommended group. It will be more than worth the cover price of this book.

VACCINES

- Pneumococcal vaccine will protect against twenty-three different strains of *Streptococcus pneumonaie,* the most common culprit in bacterial pneumonia.
- Influenza vaccine will protect against the flu, which often is the trigger to development of bacterial pneumonia.

ANTIVIRAL DRUGS

- May be used in high-risk people who develop influenza to reduce the chance of developing a secondary bacterial pneumonia.

NUTRITIONAL THERAPY

- Intravenous fluids are provided if hospitalization is needed.
- If eating is possible, light meals of soup, cereal, and puddings will provide calories, nutrients, and fluids.

HYDROTHERAPY

- When air is cold & dry, portable room humidifiers can ease breathing in heavily congested lungs.

ADDITIONAL OPTIONS

- Oxygen may be needed via nasal prongs.
- In severe cases, a mechanical respirator can provide assisted breathing and oxygen until the patient is strong enough and can "effectively" breathe on his or her own.
- Bronchodilators can be inhaled in a nebulized stream.
- Postural drainage—respiratory therapists can lightly pound the back to break up mucus.

VIRAL PNEUMONIA

Probably 20 to 30 percent of pneumonias are caused by viruses. The most common culprits are the influenza viruses. Other offenders are the adenoviruses and the Coxsackie viruses, both of which usually cause colds. Another well-known culprit is the respiratory syncytial virus, RSV, which causes pneumonia primarily in small children.

Symptoms of Viral Pneumonia

Viral pneumonias do not arrive as dramatically as those caused by bacteria. They start with chills, fever, headache, and loss of appetite, much like the symptoms of the flu virus that they are. But within three to four days, a dry cough begins, followed by shortness of breath.

Diagnosis of Viral Pneumonia

The X-ray of viral pneumonia has a distinct appearance (see Illustration on page 146). Rather than producing the clearly defined areas of infection seen in bacterial pneumonia, viral pneumonia usually produces diffuse small patches over both lungs. The fluid remains in the tissues rather than accumulating in the alveoli.

Impact of the Infection

The virus infects the cilia-topped columnar cells that transport mucus out of the airways. The cells become enlarged and cilia cannot sweep the airways clean. Mucus builds up, producing cough and inflammation. Viruses replicate inside cells, and then are released to infect other areas. As the virus reproduces, it actually destroys cells, causing fever, chills, and swelling of the airways.

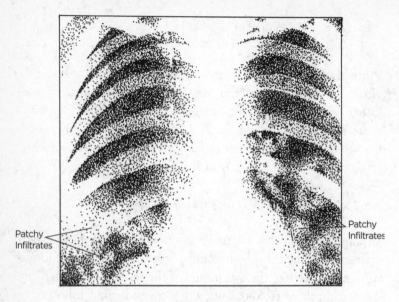

Patchy
Infiltrates

Patchy
Infiltrates

VIRAL PNEUMONIA

Preventing Viral Pneumonia

With viral pneumonia the best offense is a good defense. Follow recommendations to lower the risk of catching a cold.
Wash your hands frequently and stay away from crowds during the height of the cold season. To protect yourself from the
viral pneumonia caused by the flu, simply make sure you line up
for your annual flu shot. It is a highly effective way of preventing both influenza and viral pneumonia, both of which can be
painful and exhausting.

Treatment Issues

Viral pneumonias do not respond to the antibiotics used to
treat bacterial pneumonia. If the disease is serious enough to
warrant hospitalization, treatment usually centers on support.

If breathing is difficult, we will provide oxygen. Doctors are now using antivirals such as Tamiflu and Relenza that can both prevent and lessen the impact of both influenza and viral pneumonia if caught early. These drugs are either given orally or inhaled and taken for five to seven days.

TREATMENT PLAN: VIRAL PNEUMONIA

ANTIHISTAMINE

• Prescribed if upper airways are congested.

DECONGESTANT

• Prescribed if sinus and ears are congested.

ANTI-INFLAMMATORY

• Aspirin, acetaminophen, or ibuprofen are prescribed to control fever, aches.

QUELLING THE COUGH

• Codeine may be used to reduce chest pain and relieve cough.

ANTIBIOTICS

• Not prescribed unless there are early signs of a secondary bacterial infection (e.g., a rise in fever).

VACCINES

• Because viral pneumonia is usually part of influenza, an annual flu shot will prevent both the flu and an associated viral pneumonia.

ANTIVIRAL DRUGS

- If symptoms of pneumonia appear early during influenza, physicians may prescribe antivirals such as Relenza or Tamiflu to reduce viral impact. If symptoms of pneumonia appear more than forty-eight hours after flu has developed, antivirals are usually not indicated.

NUTRITIONAL THERAPY

- If your viral pneumonia requires hospitalization, nutrition may be provided parenterally if illness is prolonged.
- If you can eat and swallow comfortably, diet should be light, such as easily digested soups, Jell-O, and scrambled eggs.

HYDROTHERAPY

- A portable room humidifier can soften hardened mucus in the lungs.

ADDITIONAL SUPPORT

- Oxygen supplied through nasal prongs can assist infected lungs.
- If respiration is especially labored, mechanical support may be needed until the infection is brought under better control.

Complications of Viral Pneumonia

The most common complication in viral pneumonia is the development of a secondary bacterial pneumonia. The fluid and mucus that accumulate in the airways are a perfect growing medium for the bacteria that routinely live in the upper airways. It is important that you and your physician be aware of any change in your symptoms that could signal the arrival of a second form of pneumonia. These would include an increase in fever, chest pain, and the development of a wet cough that brings up rusty-colored sputum.

MYCOPLASMA PNEUMONIA

The third type of pneumonia is known as atypical or *mycoplasma* pneumonia. Tom, whom we met earlier in this chapter, had this form of pneumonia, which is usually seen in younger, healthier adults, and older children. It is caused by mycoplasma, the smallest living organisms, which are midway in development between a virus and a bacteria.

Mycoplasma are surface parasites: they cling to the top of cell membranes and rarely invade tissues or the bloodstream, but their attachments lead to cell damage and cell death. Mycoplasma pneumonia can cause widespread, albeit usually mild, pneumonia that is transmitted by person-to-person contact. In fact, it is the only pneumonia that you catch. Popularly called walking pneumonia, outbreaks of mycoplasma pneumonia are common among college students and military recruits, all living in close quarters in dormitories and barracks.

Mycoplasma pneumonia may start with coldlike symptoms, chills, and fever. The most characteristic symptom is a lingering cough that produces almost violent coughing spasms with little or no mucus. It can go on for months and make victims like Tom feel exhausted.

On X-ray, mycoplasma pneumonia looks similar to that seen in viral pneumonia. The lungs have small patches of infection over both lungs. We can also use blood analysis called serology to check for antibodies to mycoplasma. Your body produces these antibodies in response to mycoplasma infection. A rising level of antibodies is a clear sign that this organism has caused disease in the body. Antibody levels identify mycoplasma especially well because the disease is slow and lingering, giving time for titers or levels of the antibody to build. A combination of history, X-ray, and repeated blood tests can accurately identify mycoplasma pneumonia.

TREATMENT PLAN: MYCOPLASMA "WALKING" PNEUMONIA

ANTIHISTAMINE

• Generally not prescribed.

DECONGESTANT

• Generally not prescribed.

ANTI-INFLAMMATORY

• Acetaminophen or ibuprofen can be prescribed to relieve fever.

QUELLING THE COUGH

• Cough syrups with guaifenesin can be used to loosen hard, dry mucus.
• Cough medication with codeine can be ordered to relieve exhausting cough (a frequent symptom of mycoplasma pneumonia).

Treatment Issues

Mycoplasma pneumonia does not respond to the penicillin family of antibiotics. In fact, it is often the failure of a patient to respond to what is felt to be the first-choice treatment for bacterial pneumonias that suggests to doctors that they are dealing with mycoplasma. Fortunately, mycoplasma can be brought under control with newer broad-spectrum antibiotics such as erythromycin or Tequin.

ANTIBIOTICS

- Macrolides such as Biaxin or Zithromax, tetracyclines, or Levaquin are the antibiotics of choice. They need to be taken for seven to ten days, but occasionally longer.

VACCINES

- None available.

ANTIVIRAL DRUGS

- Not applicable.

NUTRITIONAL THERAPY

- Normal meals.
- Hot tea and chicken soup will temporarily relieve feelings of congestion.

HYDROTHERAPY

- Hot shower in the morning will help lungs breathe easier.
- In cold, dry weather, a portable room humidifier will loosen mucus in the airways.

Complications of Mycoplasma Pneumonia

Mycoplasma pneumonia is usually a long but uncomplicated illness. When it affects older people or those with underlying health problems, a problem with the blood called *hemolytic anemia* has been known to develop. For reasons that are not clear, antibodies produced in response to the mycoplasma attach themselves to the red blood cells and destroy them. Symptoms of hemolytic anemia include pallor, fatigue, and shortness of breath. It can successfully be treated with a combination of steroids and blood transfusions.

Preventing Mycoplasma Pneumonia

There is no vaccine for mycoplasma pneumonia. It is spread by droplets and infected materials from person to person much in the same way that influenza is transmitted. Limiting the infection depends on recognizing that an outbreak is happening in a community and taking measures to isolate and treat those who are infected. Appropriate hygiene strategies, such as hand washing and not handling potentially infected objects, will ensure that you don't come in contact with infected materials.

CHAPTER 9

INFLUENZA—THE COLD'S
EVIL TWIN

At fifty-seven, Peggy Sue Coopersmith had been the manager for a team of female wrestlers, a radio talk show host, and the owner of arguably the best coffee bar in Brooklyn. Coop, as her friends called her, was proud of her ongoing good health and cheerfully ignored my recommendations for an annual flu shot. After a weeklong bout of cough and high fever that left her, in her own words, "too exhausted to talk," Coop dragged herself into the ER, convinced she had a rare deadly disease. She was stunned to hear that she had the flu, the same flu that was affecting millions of Americans across the United States that winter. Although she had ignored the flu vaccine recommendations for most of her adult life, the impact of this experience convinced her to be first in line for "the jab" in the years that followed.

Like a cold, influenza is caused by a virus, but the similarities are superficial. Along with Sunday football and Thanksgiving turkeys, influenza makes an annual appearance every fall. In the United States, the flu annually affects up to 60 million children and adults, causes up to two hundred thousand people to be hospitalized, and is fatal to more than twenty thousand people.

Influenza—the Last Great Plague

The scourge of smallpox, measles, and bubonic plague have long been controlled by the development of vaccines, antibiotics, and new public health policies. But despite all the advances in science, the flu continues to affect hundreds of millions of people worldwide each year. When the flu affects large numbers of people in a community, it is said to be an epidemic. When the flu affects people all over the world, it is called a pandemic.

Over the centuries, there have been notable outbreaks of flu. The first epidemic was described by the great Greek physician Hippocrates, in 412 B.C. Physicians in sixteenth-century Europe described outbreaks of severe, but not necessarily fatal, respiratory infections. Over the next two hundred years, fifteen pandemics of severe influenza caused disease and death. However, it was the influenza pandemic of 1899 that had a disturbingly high death rate. It began in eastern Russia, close to the Chinese border. As it spread across the world, it caused new levels of chaos heretofore unknown with the influenza virus. In many places, 40 to 50 percent of the population fell seriously ill. Many researchers believe that the genetic changes in the virus of the 1899 epidemic were the basis of what became the influenza pandemic of 1918.

This influenza pandemic of 1918, also known as the Spanish flu, is the benchmark outbreak by which we define influenza today. Over two years, it affected over 200 million people and killed an estimated 21 to 50 million worldwide. In the United States, five hundred thousand adults and children died from the Spanish flu. Unlike in other flu epidemics, where the elderly succumb, young adults had extraordinarily high death rates. In fact, 50 percent of all deaths were in young, healthy adults, aged twenty to forty.

Looking back at the health records of the time, in the two previous years there had been scattered, sporadic outbreaks of a severe influenza. In the spring of 1918, American troops were mobilizing to join the Western Front in World War I. In March, influenza broke out in a Kansas military camp, and though severe, most of the soldiers survived. Within weeks, the flu spread to thousands of young men crowded together in military camps and troop ships. Soon it infected civilians, affecting tens of thousands. By early summer, the flu had spread worldwide, and as it traveled, it seemed to gather strength. In August, the disease turned deadly. Young, strong men became ill and died within hours.

Pneumonia is usually an occasional complication of the flu, but in the 1918 influenza, one in ten people with the flu developed pneumonia. By the time the pandemic ended, the virus had killed 2 percent of the world's population. Normally, the flu virus attacks only the respiratory system, and this virus did this with unprecedented speed and violence. The lungs of its victims were literally drowned in water and debris and were almost completely destroyed.

In addition, the 1918 flu virus underwent enough of a genetic change to attack organs all over the body. Frequently, it attacked and destroyed the liver and kidneys. Stomach muscles ruptured and hemorrhaged. Many who survived never fully recovered. There was an unprecedented increase in chronic endocarditis, a usually rare heart disease. Others suffered permanent neurological damage. In the fifteen years after the 1918 outbreak ended, many of survivors developed a form of encephalitis that left them in a lifelong coma. Doctors suspect that this form of sleeping sickness, movingly described by Oliver Sacks in his book *Awakenings,* was due to the impact of the 1918 influenza virus on the brains, or neurological systems of the survivors.

Fortunately, doctors believe that even if a similar virus appeared today, increased disease surveillance and medical advances in prevention and treatment would prevent a repetition of the worst influenza pandemic in history. Keep in mind that in

SIMPLE SOLUTIONS FOR A BIG PAIN

These characteristic aches are caused by the flood of inflammatory agents that the body produces as part of its defense system. Anti-inflammatory compounds, such as acetaminophen, ibuprofen, and aspirin block the release of these agents and contribute to temporary relief. For details on how these compounds work, see chapter 3.

1918 we did not even know that influenza was caused by a virus. There was no immunization, little or no supportive care, no oxygen, and no antibiotics or antivirals to treat the disease and its complications.

The worldwide death and suffering from this influenza pandemic spurred politicians and the military to support research to prevent a repeat of the chaos. In 1933, an Iowa-based virologist, Richard Shope, isolated the virus. By the time the armies had mobilized again for World War II, troops had received an effective influenza vaccine.

Symptoms of the Flu

The flu starts suddenly. One minute you feel fine, the next you have a headache. Within a few hours you feel acutely ill with fever, body aches, and exhaustion. A harsh dry cough begins within twenty-four hours. Eyes can be sensitive to light and nausea is not uncommon. To add insult to injury, you can also have coldlike congestion and sneezing. Severe body aches and exhaustion are key markers of this infection. You may feel too weak to get out of bed and find it painful even to turn over.

The acute phase of the flu lasts three to five days. If symptoms continue or the fever goes up, it is likely that a secondary bronchitis, pneumonia, or sinusitis has developed. In fact, at least 60 percent of the flu is complicated by bronchitis.

Is It a Cold or Flu?

By definition a cold is an upper respiratory infection and affects the nose, throat, ears, and eyes. Symptoms start slowly and build up over twenty-four hours. In a simple cold, fever is mild, and while you may feel uncomfortable, you can carry on with work and school.

Influenza is considered a lower respiratory disorder that affects the throat and large airways of the lungs. Classic flu symptoms arrive suddenly and intensively. You may feel so awful and exhausted that all you can do is sleep. A body-racking cough begins within a day, adding to your general discomfort.

But cold and flu viruses don't always follow neat guidelines. A particularly vicious cold virus, especially in smokers or people with underlying lung problems such as asthma, can produce severe symptoms. Similarly, a traditional flu can be accompanied by sneezing and stuffy nose. Additionally, if you have some resistance to the flu virus or it is the milder influenza B or C virus, the disease can resemble a heavy cold.

If you are a healthy adult under age sixty, less aggressive infections will be short-lived and respond well to rest, fluids, and medications to relieve symptoms.

When the symptoms are severe and if you are over sixty, recognizing the flu early can be important to preventing potentially serious complications. If flu is recognized in the first forty-eight hours of infection, antivirals (such as Tamiflu) can reduce the severity and duration of symptoms.

The similarity of symptoms between a cold and flu can make diagnosis difficult, even for a doctor. To find the right answer, three questions can provide clues:

TIMING OF SYMPTOMS. One of the best clues are the characteristics of the first symptoms. When sneezing and a scratchy throat announce the beginnings of a problem, the cold virus is probably the culprit. If your first signs are fever, headache, and exhaustion, you're probably another statistic for the National Influenza Surveillance System.

SEASON OF THE SYMPTOMS. The cold season runs from September to March, but colds can occur at any time of the year. The influenza season is clearly seasonal with a peak from November to February. A respiratory infection in the spring and summer months is likely a cold. If you fall ill at the height of the flu season, odds are that you are suffering from influenza.

SEVERITY OF SYMPTOMS. A cold can be annoying and depressing, but you still have the energy to complain. In a flu you often feel too miserable to talk. The fever, body aches, and bone-jarring cough make you weak and ill. Once you have had a full-blown flu, it is likely that you will know when it has struck again.

Causes of Influenza

Influenza is caused by a unique and fascinating virus. The three types of flu virus are designated A, B, and C. Type A is the most serious and is the cause of pandemics or worldwide epidemics. It is the only one that occurs both in animals and humans. Type B causes epidemics less frequently, usually affects only children, and produces less severe disease. Type C is usually not a part of the influenza outbreaks.

It is believed that the natural reservoir of the flu virus live harmlessly in the digestive tracts of waterfowl such as ducks and geese, particularly those that live in the Far East. Most of the new widespread strains of influenza start in China, such as the Asian flu of 1957, the Hong Kong flu of 1968, and the Fujian of 2003. In China, where densely crowded people live in close proximity to large populations of birds, pigs, and other animals, the opportunity for cross-infection between human and animal is always present. Epidemiologists, therefore, concentrate a great deal of effort on monitoring flulike illnesses in China each year, to identify the new strains that are causing them.

Both types A and B tend to change their genetic structure each year. When the change is slight, it is called antigenic drift. When the change is big, it is known as antigenic shift. When you recover from a case of the flu, you develop antibodies to that virus. If that virus appears again, you will have antibodies to protect you from infection. When the antigenic drift is small, your existing antibodies may protect you against the newer form of the virus or, at the least, lessen the severity of your next infection with that strain. More usually, the drift in genetic makeup will make your existing antibodies ineffective. As a result, each year the flu vaccine needs to contain new antigens that more closely resemble new forms of the influenza virus.

The genetic changes also alter the types of illness that develop in your community. Some years, the genetic drifts cause mild disease. Other years, they increase risk of pneumonia, nausea, or even mental depression. In most cases, a virus is normally specific for a single species. For example, Newcastle disease kills entire flocks of chickens, but does not cause illness in humans. By the same token, mumps or chicken pox, which affect children, are not passed on to household pets.

By contrast, the influenza virus not only affects birds, pigs, and horses, but humans as well. And as the influenza virus moves through different species, it changes characteristics. Scientists believe that the deadly 1918–19 influenza epidemic that killed up to 50 million people worldwide began in a Kansas military camp where pigs infected with an influenza passed the disease to the troops stationed there. The genetic shift of this swine flu led to a virus deadly for human beings. While genetic drifts occur each year, it is the changes that occur when this virus passes from animal to human that produce severe killer viruses.

THE ARRIVAL OF THE AVIAN FLU

In 1997, an outbreak of a deadly type of influenza was traced to infection from chickens. All of the forty-five children and adults stricken caught the flu directly from contact with these birds. It was especially troubling that 75 percent of the people affected died. Because the disease was caught from chickens, millions of birds were destroyed to stop its spread. The only good news was that the virus was not spread from person to person. What doctors fear now is that the genetic material from the bird virus will some-day combine with genetic material from the human virus, some-thing that influenza viruses are capable of doing, to form a deadly form of influenza that can be spread through the air from one person to another.

The Influenza Early Warning System

The World Health Organization (WHO) coordinates the international influenza surveillance program. It works with a world-wide network of one hundred laboratories. These centers are constantly vigilant in isolating and examining blood samples for new viruses. Any unusual organisms or results are sent to the WHO collecting centers. At the end of winter, vaccine specialists meet to decide which of the new strains should be used in the new flu vaccine.

Under an electron microscope, the flu virus looks like a weapon developed by a mad scientist. It is a round ball covered with two types of "spikes"—the hemagglutinin (H) and the neuraminidase (N) (see Illustration on page 161). Changes in these two spikes cause variants of the virus that result in pandemics. The type of influenza virus from the 1918 epidemic is designated H1N1. Since 1918, there have been several major genetic shifts. The next major shift resulted in the 1957 Asian flu (H2N2), which took the lives of seventy thousand Ameri-

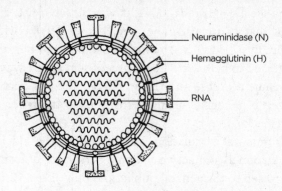

Neuraminidase (N)

Hemagglutinin (H)

RNA

THE INFLUENZA VIRUS

cans. A decade later, the Hong Kong flu (H3N2) caused a severe infection that killed almost forty thousand Americans. Worldwide, the combined mortality for Asian and Hong Kong flu was 1 million men, women, and children.

Another influenza pandemic is long overdue, and any sign that it might be starting sends doctors and public health officials into a justified panic. In 1976, a small outbreak of a severe flu occurred at Fort Dix, New Jersey. During a cold, wet January, a group of new recruits arrived at the base. Within a few days, normally healthy young men began to appear at the infirmary. At first the doctors thought it was just a bad cold, but one doctor with the New Jersey Department of Health was suspicious. He sent blood samples to the Centers for Disease Control to see if they could identify the virus.

As the doctors waited for the results, more and more soldiers continued to flood into the infirmary. In early February, Private David Lewis, although achy and feverish, joined his fellow recruits on a routine five-mile march. Young and in otherwise excellent health, Private Lewis collapsed during the march. In less than twenty-four hours, he was dead of an overwhelming pneumonia. A few days later, the CDC reported that a number of recruits, including the late Private Lewis, had a form of swine flu. Designated H1N1, it was closely related to the deadly flu that had caused the pandemic of 1918. It had been more than fifty years since swine flu had infected humans, and now it seemed to be back. The discovery sent shock waves through government offices and research labs. The prospect of another swine flu pandemic changed forever our approach to influenza vaccination.

In 1976, influenza inoculation was limited to the elderly, health care personnel, and active military personnel. Vaccination was a hard sell to the general public, and only about 12–16 million Americans received the vaccine each year.

In 1957, although scientists knew that the Asian flu (H2N2) was coming, the government did not call for a national vaccination program. Without a guarantee of use, pharmaceutical companies would not make large amounts of the vaccine. When the Asian flu arrived, seventy-thousand people died, and manufacturers were left with millions of vaccine doses they could not sell. Vaccination programs did not fare much better when the Hong Kong flu struck in 1968 and almost forty-thousand people died.

Doctors and virologists had been warning about the arrival of another pandemic when in 1976 swine flu appeared at Fort Dix, affecting more than five hundred personnel on the base. President Gerald Ford called for the first national program to vaccinate all Americans. At first everything went well as tens of thousands of Americans began to receive the swine flu vaccine in early fall of 1977.

Soon after the immunization program began, however, two issues appeared. For reasons no one could fathom, the swine flu did not spread—and the cases at Fort Dix remained isolated events. That was the good news. The bad news? Reports began to surface of a serious neurological problem, called Guillian-Barre syndrome, that was affecting people who had received the vaccine. By the time 46 million Americans had received their shot, five hundred people had developed the debilitating disease and twenty-seven died. The vaccination program was suspended in a torrent of controversy and finger-pointing.

Problems with the vaccine sparked a federal investigation. A blue-ribbon panel concluded that despite the problems, it had been the right decision to pursue influenza inoculation. The panel noted that while it is impossible to predict which strains will take hold and which won't, if the swine flu had exploded, millions of lives could have been lost. Other experts suggested that the unusual level of neurological complications were a reflection of the virulence of the swine flu virus and not a problem with the vaccine. Despite these reassurances, the influenza vaccination program suffered a loss of public confidence that has taken decades to overcome.

In the fall of 2003, a severe early flu struck six thousand people in Colorado, killing twenty-five children. Public health officials, already concerned with the virulence and rapid spread of the outbreak, were even more concerned when the culprit turned out to be the newly identified Fujian strain (H3N3). Even more troubling, the flu vaccine for the year was ready for distribution but did not include this clearly powerful strain. A year earlier, influenza experts were aware that the new strain had appeared in China, but could not get the virus into production for the following year. They decided to include the closely related Panama H3N3, which was already in current vaccine production. The strategy didn't work out as well as they had hoped.

The 2003 vaccine was only 40–60 percent effective in conferring immunity to influenza. By contrast, the annual flu vaccine is characteristically 70–80 percent protective. The following year, 2004, the vaccine contained the once-feared Fujian strain, but by then it had been eclipsed by a milder flu strain.

The concerns about the genetic changes of the swine and Fujian flu pale beside the concerns about the latest variant known as H5N1. Normally this strain affects only birds, but in

1997 it infected forty-five people in different parts of Southeast Asia. It caused an overwhelming infection that was fatal to thirty-five children and adults—a mortality rate of 75 percent. Given that the mortality rate for the 1918 epidemic was 2 percent, doctors are right to be worried. To some researchers this outbreak had all the earmarks of the influenza doomsday scenario, where an animal flu strain changes into a deadly form that infects humans. To date almost everyone infected became ill by direct contact with chickens. Public health officals in Asia responded by killing millions of birds where the virus could be detected in the flocks.

This strategy may have prevented a widespread outbreak, but the avian flu has continued to spread across the Far East. To date it has been identified in victims in Laos, Vietnam, Thailand, Cambodia, Indonesia, and Malaysia. In only a few cases did it spread by contact with an infected family member. What doctors fear is that the H5N1 virus will continue to mutate and become able to be spread from person to person. Many experts are concerned that our current viral detection and vaccine production techniques are not up to the challenge of the avian flu.

Reverse Genetics

The early warning system of identifying new viral strains has been used for more than sixty years. While it has worked well, it is also a risky race against time to identify every year the dominant virus strains, pick the right ones to include in the vaccine, then produce and distribute influenza protection by the next flu season. To be more proactive, virologists have been working on a technique known as *reverse genetics*. Instead of waiting anxiously for the next natural and dangerous variation, reverse genetics engineers an anticipated strain, but includes less virulent genetic codes. The lab-made virus can be used to safely produce an effective vaccine against a potential killer.

Reverse genetics are now being used to develop an effective vaccine against the dreaded avian H5N1.

So far the work has had a slow start. Rather than being created in a test tube (as with reverse genetics), influenza virus is grown in fertilized eggs and harvested to produce a vaccine. Unfortunately, the bird virus kills the eggs before sufficient viral levels can develop. This new type of virus has forced researchers to look for new ways to work with influenza virus. The egg-based vaccine is an old technology, and the necessity of finding a new approach will, in the long run, benefit vaccine development in general.

Transmission of Influenza

The flu virus is spread through the air by droplets from infected people. You actually start shedding the flu virus twenty-four hours before symptoms develop, so you can spread influenza without even knowing you're sick. Once symptoms develop (usually within two days of exposure), you are contagious for another five days. People who do not seem to catch the flu during an epidemic often have a subclinical case; that is, an infection with few or mild symptoms. It is estimated that four times as many people have this "silent" flu as those who develop full-blown symptoms. However, people infected with this symptomless flu can also spread infection, and this is one reason why the infection first seems to break out sporadically, then suddenly explodes in large numbers in the community.

Normally, people infected with a respiratory disease feel too sick to continue their normal activities. But doctors believe that this large number of symptomless flu victims contributes to the rapid, worldwide spread of influenza once the virus arrives. The flu virus can also linger for hours in the air, waiting for someone to make contact. It can seemingly travel miles in the air. Outbreaks have been reported between isolated farms, with no human contact, and yet the animals at both farms became in-fected. Sailors on ships, who have been out at sea for weeks, spontaneously came down with influenza after passing miles off the coast where influenza affected the land communities.

It is no coincidence that flu season is accompanied by cold, windy weather. Chilly temperatures mean that people spend more time crowded together indoors with their windows shut in their homes, offices, and apartments, raising the viral load in the air.

The cold, gray skies and short days of winter also seem to con-tribute to the spread of the flu. Sunlight and warmth are lethal to the virus. Some researchers suggest the cold, dark windy nights may spread the virus from one community to another. While re-peated experiments have shown that cold, damp weather does not cause increased susceptibility to colds and flu, this type of weather may increase transmission of influenza, supporting the age-old connection of illness with cold, winter weather.

The Impact on the Body

The influenza virus usually confines itself to the trachea and bronchi (see Illustration on page 15). Molecular biologists have shown that cells in the throat and bronchi have receptor sites that bind with the hemagglutinin spikes that the virus uses to enter the cell.

When the cold virus attacks a cell, it replicates rapidly in-side, but leaves the cell intact. You develop annoying symp-toms, but generally mild enough for you to continue with your daily activities. By contrast, when the flu virus replicates rap-idly, thousands of new virus particles burst out, destroying the cell. In addition to the release of millions of new viruses, the dying cells spill inflammatory proteins throughout the body. The extreme cellular damage leads to a high level of cytokines, which produces the exhaustion and high fever of the flu. It's lit-

WHEN A FLU VIRUS EXTENDS ITS REACH

Normally the flu virus confines its attack to the cells of the throat and large airways. In smokers or in people with asthma, already fragile airways can come under direct viral attack. When the virus invades the alveoli or the interstitial lung tissue, a simple flu becomes viral pneumonia. Key signs of viral pneumonia are chest pain and shortness of breath. Changes in the genetic makeup of the flu virus can also extend the variety of organs that are infected. In the 1918 pandemic, the virus attacked the liver, kidney, heart, and brain.

tle wonder you feel so much worse with the flu since aches, pains, and fevers are directly proportional to the amount of inflammatory compounds in the body. The cough, which is arguably the worst part of the flu, develops when the inflammatory compounds from dead and dying cells irritate the nerves in the throat and airways, triggering the cough reflex.

Diagnosis of Influenza

Diagnosis is usually made on the basis of the symptoms and the season. If the flu is in full swing between November and February, and the symptoms are fever over 101, cough, and exhaustion, most doctors feel comfortable with a diagnosis of influenza. If your symptoms are especially severe, such as a fever over 103 or shortness of breath, or if you develop flulike symptoms in the early spring and summer months, your physician may send a blood sample to try to identify the virus that is causing your problems. But in general, the diagnosis is made without laboratory testing.

Complications of Influenza

Complications are usually considered an occasional problem in most respiratory diseases. But with influenza, it is more likely than not that additional problems will develop:

INFLUENZA PLUS BRONCHITIS. Acute bronchitis is noted in at least 60 percent of people with influenza. Exposure to cigarette smoke and air pollution seem to increase the risk of developing bronchitis with influenza. In addition, if you have underlying diseases such as asthma or emphysema, it is almost guaranteed that you will develop additional pulmonary problems.

In the usual course of a flu, fever, sore throat, and body aches start to subside within three days. When the virus invades the trachea, a burning chest pain may develop when you cough or even breathe. If fever starts rising again and the cough becomes more severe, you have probably developed a case of acute viral bronchitis. If greenish mucus is produced or the fever continues to be over 101, bacterial infection may have begun, and antibiotics may be prescribed.

INFLUENZA PLUS PNEUMONIA. Pneumonia is one of the most serious complications of influenza. In some cases, the influenza virus directly infects the airways. Clear symptoms of the appearance of viral pneumonia include high fever and severe shortness of breath, which develops within three to four days after coming down with the initial flu. Shortness of breath can be so severe that oxygen support may be required. In older people, especially those with underlying health problems, viral pneumonia can rapidly be fatal. Influenza can also develop into a severe bacterial pneumonia.

If high fever or shortness of breath or the cough becomes more severe, doctors suspect that bacterial colonization of the lungs may have developed. Bacterial pneumonia develops when the influenza virus sufficiently damages the surface of the airways so that they can no longer clear themselves of mucus. The buildup of debris leads to growth in the lungs of pneumonia-causing bacteria. Bacterial pneumonia is announced by shaking chills, a rise in fever, chest pain, shortness of breath, and a rust-colored sputum. It is possible to have both viral and bacterial pneumonias at the same time. Mortality for patients hospitalized with influenza complicated by pneumonia can be as high as 50 percent. Although it is generally most serious in the elderly during influenza pandemics, 50 percent of deaths occur in people younger than sixty-five.

REYE'S SYNDROME. Reye's syndrome is an acute illness that causes swelling of the brain and severe liver damage. It primarily affects young children after viral infections such as influenza or chicken pox. In 1982, the surgeon general issued an advisory to parents against using aspirin in children with chicken pox or flulike illnesses due to their link with Reye's syndrome.

Prevention of Influenza

The flu and its potential complications can be prevented by two widely available, inexpensive, and safe vaccines. The yearly flu vaccine contains three different strains of the flu virus. Each year, new strains of influenza develop, and the annual vaccine is designed to protect you against the newly established strains. In 2004, the recommendations for vaccinations were broadened to cover more children and adults who were at higher risk for complications. For a complete list of people who should receive vaccination, see page 41.

Generally, those who should be vaccinated include anyone over fifty, residents of nursing homes, children under twenty-three months, adults or children over twenty-three months with diabetes, heart disease, chronic lung disease, or those with an impaired immune system, family members and caregivers of high-risk people, doctors and health care workers, pregnant women in the second and third trimesters, and children under eighteen on chronic aspirin therapy.

The Shortage of the Vaccine

In 2004, new recommendations extending the at-risk group for influenza came out, and that year also saw a critical shortage of flu vaccine. Because of the way flu vaccine was bought and regulated, it discouraged pharmaceutical companies from producing this much needed preventive tool (see chapter 3). By 2004, all of our flu vaccine came from just two companies: Chiron, located in England, and Aventis, located in the United States.

An accident happened in production of the flu vaccine in England, contaminating 50 million doses or half of the required doses for the United States. The outrage that followed the shortage and the recognition that this problem had been predicted for many years is going to lead to changes in the way a vaccine is produced and hopefully the way the industry is regulated.

Who Should Get the Flu Vaccine?

There are two prevailing attitudes about who should get vaccinated. The traditional approach has been to protect those at highest risk of complications—the elderly, those with underlying health problems, and young children. In terms of public health, however, immunizing high-risk people is not that effective in controlling the spread (and cost) of the disease. To that end, some influenza experts advocate widespread vaccination to increase general resistance to the virus—a concept known as herd immunity.

Here's how it works. The more people who are resistant to the virus, the less likely it is to spread. Studies have shown that half of the population needs to be vaccinated for herd immunity to develop. It has been suggested that facing so few susceptible hosts, the virus loses steam and fades away. Some even suggest that the failure of the swine flu in 1976 to become an epidemic was due to the rapid vaccination program. Although the program was stopped before everyone had been vaccinated, the vaccine had been administered to 46 million Americans, which may have been enough to produce a degree of herd immunity.

Rather than focusing on the people who are susceptible to complications, supporters of the herd immunity approach recommend vaccination of those who are most likely to spread the virus—school-age children. A single infected child can give the virus to classmates and teachers, who will then infect family members. To back up their theories, doctors point out that the elderly come in contact with far fewer people and are thus less likely to infect others. In addition, they point out while the flu vaccine is 70 to 90 percent effective in children and adults, the decreased immune response in people over age sixty-five renders the vaccine only 35 to 40 percent effective in them. In fact, a study from Britain found that the best way to lower death rates from the flu in a nursing home was to immunize the staff rather than the residents.

The new vaccination guidelines issued in 2004 cover about 100 million people, or about half of the entire population. I am an enthusiastic supporter of the flu shot and recommend everyone have it except those who have an allergy to eggs.

Pneumonia Vaccine: The Second Line of Defense

Influenza and its complication of bacterial pneumonia are a debilitating combination. Fortunately, the pneumonia vaccine will protect against twenty-three different strains of streptococcus, the most common pneumonia organism. Pneumonia vaccine is recommended for three large groups of people: all individuals over sixty-five; people over the age of two with underlying health problems such as asthma, diabetes, or heart disease; and people over two who have suppressed immunity, such as those with HIV or who are on steroids or receiving chemotherapy.

A yearly flu shot and, if indicated, a single pneumonia shot will keep your winters safer and healthier.

Treatment Issues for Influenza

The flu virus provokes release of large amounts of inflammatory compounds such as prostaglandins and interleukins, which cause fever, body aches, and exhaustion. The foundation of flu treatment starts with regular use of anti-inflammatory agents such aspirin, acetaminophen, or ibuprofen. Regular use of anti-inflammatory agents will reduce the intense discomfort of the flu. Other symptoms such as sore throat, congestion, and cough can be relieved with specific remedies.

For patients with underlying health problems such as diabetes or asthma, I can prescribe antiviral medications such as Tamiflu that block the replication of the flu virus in the body. These need to be taken within the first forty-eight hours of symptoms. After that time, the influenza viruses have produced a flood of inflammatory cytokines, and body aches and fever need to be treated directly.

Antibiotics do not control the flu virus, but they can be used if increased fever and darkening mucus indicate bronchitis has developed.

TREATMENT PLAN: INFLUENZA

ANTIHISTAMINE

- If there is sneezing and congestion, take traditional antihistamine twice a day. Sedation will not usually be a problem since you will feel too sick to work or play.

DECONGESTANT

- If there is congestion, use decongestants according to manufacturer's instructions. Use decongestant sprays for only three days to avoid rebound congestion (see page 29). If congestion continues, switch to an oral form for another four days of the acute stage of the flu.

ANTI-INFLAMMATORY

- Take acetaminophen, ibuprofen, or aspirin at the start of the flu symptoms and continue taking them every four hours for the next four to five days for fever, aches, and general fatigue.

QUELLING THE COUGH

- Cough suppressant with dextromethorphan or codeine (with prescription) as directed by label instructions.
- Lozenges with benzocaine to soothe throat pain and quiet cough reflex.

ANTIBIOTICS

- Not necessary unless you have asthma, COPD, or other underlying health problems and secondary bronchitis is suspected.
- If cough continues or increases after seven days, green phlegm is produced, or fever increases, antibiotics such Augmentin, Biaxin, or Zithromax may be prescribed.

VACCINES

- Make your annual flu shot as much part of a fall tradition as the Halloween pumpkin.
- If you meet the guidelines for the lifetime pneumonia shot (see page 171), make sure you have this shot that offers a lifetime of protection.

ANTIVIRAL THERAPY

- Starting within forty-eight hours of symptoms, Tamiflu or Relenza twice a day for five to seven days may shorten the length of illness.

NUTRITIONAL THERAPY

- Light meals of eggs, toast, hot cereal, soups, Jell-O, ice cream, sherbet, and pudding.
- Three to four cups of hot and iced tea daily.
- One glass of orange juice daily.
- Avoid high-fat foods such as fried food, pizza, and salty snacks.

HYDROTHERAPY

- Saline gargle two or three times a day to relieve sore throat pain.

SUPPLEMENTS

- None indicated helpful.

CHAPTER 10

THE SNEEZING YEARS—COLDS AND FLU IN CHILDHOOD

The *Good Doctor's Guide to Colds and Flu* is focused on providing health information to adults. This chapter is not meant to be a comprehensive guide to children's respiratory illnesses, but there are important differences in symptoms and treatments between children and adults, and I want parents to be aware of them. The first six medical problems discussed in this chapter are commonly seen in both adults and children. These sections point out key differences between the two groups. Issues not covered in this chapter are similar for both parents and child. The three final respiratory illnesses I discuss in this chapter are specific to infants and children. All aspects of the diseases from diagnosis to prevention are covered.

COLDS IN CHILDHOOD

Sniffles and sneezes are as much a part of childhood as bike riding and birthday parties. Colds are responsible for 20 million missed days of school in the United States. While in the womb and at birth, your child receives antibodies through the placenta. These usually remain active for three to six months. Children usually get their first cold at four months, when mom's antibodies have disappeared. Children typically get six to eight colds per year, and each cold lasts for ten to fourteen days. So if you feel that your child always has a cold or sniffles, you're not far from wrong. The more children in the family, the more colds occur. In many households, boys get more colds than girls, but moms catch colds more frequently than dads.

Symptoms of a Cold in Childhood

Cold symptoms tend to be more severe in children. In children under the age of one, gastrointestinal problems, such as diarrhea and spitting up, can accompany sneezes and sniffles. In children up to age twelve, cold symptoms may routinely include sore throat, irritability, difficulty sleeping, decreased appetite, and swollen glands.

Transmission of Colds

Incubation time for a cold is one to five days after exposure to a virus. Children can actually be contagious one or two days before symptoms develop. Because they have already "shared" their cold with their classmates, it is not necessary or even helpful to keep them home until they are symptom-free. It won't stop spreading the colds, and your children might miss months of school.

Complications of a Cold in Childhood

Children tend to develop different complications from adults. Up to 80 percent of youngsters with colds develop some degree of earache. Children's eustachian tubes are narrow and horizontal to the ears, leading to blockage and fluid backup. In adults, the eustachian tubes are proportionately wider and tilt downward to promote drainage. Earaches are so common in children that they are covered in depth in this chapter on page 192.

Bronchitis is far less common in children, and sinusitis usually occurs only in children with underlying allergies. A cold that lingers past fourteen days, accompanied by cloudy, thick mucus, may indicate a bacterial infection has developed in the sinus cavities. In children with asthma, a cold can provoke a full-blown attack. In fact, it is estimated that at least 50 percent of asthmatic episodes in children begin with a simple cold or flu.

Pneumonia may develop in young children with underlying health problems. Premature infants, children with heart disease or birth defects, are at a higher risk for a cold to progress to viral or bacterial pneumonia. If a baby or small child develops rapid breathing during a cold, it could indicate pneumonia, and it is a signal to call your pediatrician immediately.

Treatment Issues of Colds in Childhood

There are important differences in the management of colds in infants and children compared to adults. Some treatment options need to be avoided, while new choices can be of benefit. Aspirin should never be given to children under age eighteen because of its link to a serious, potentially fatal complication known as Reye's syndrome. This acute illness causes swelling of the brain and severe liver damage. It primarily affects young children after viral infections such as influenza and chicken pox. It begins with vomiting, irritability, and confusion that rapidly progresses to coma.

Reye's syndrome was first identified in 1963 in Australia. National Reye's surveillance was established in the United States in 1973, during an anticipated influenza outbreak. In the decade that followed, doctors recognized a link between the use of aspirin in viral illness and an increased risk of Reye's. In

1980, a total of 555 cases were reported nationwide. In 1982, the surgeon general issued an advisory that warned parents about using aspirin in children with chicken pox or flulike illnesses. By 1985–86, just under one hundred cases were reported. As more parents recognized the dangers of aspirin in this situation, the incidence of Reye's continued to drop. Since 1997, no more than two cases a year have been reported.

Although Reye's has not been linked to colds, it is often hard to differentiate between the two viral illnesses, especially in the early stages. To avoid potential problems, most pediatricians caution parents against using aspirin in childhood illnesses. To control fever and body aches, use acetaminophen or ibuprofen that is specifically formulated for children. Dosages of medication in children are based on age and/or body weight. The recommended dosage of acetaminophen is 10mg/2.2 pounds of body weight. For example, an infant of less than twelve pounds should take no more than 40 mg of acetaminophen, up to four times a day. A school-age child who weighs between thirty-six and forty-seven pounds can take 230 mg, up to four times a day. Follow the manufacturer's guidelines on the product package for the right dosage, and don't exceed recommendations.

Antihistamines should not be used in children under age six. They tend to make children sleepy and are best used at bedtime in older children. Pseudoephedrine decongestants, which can increase blood pressure, are not recommended for children under age six. To relieve congestion, you can gently suction the mucus with a nasal bulb, which is available in pharmacies. Alternatively, you can put three drops of saline nasal wash into each nostril. For children over age six, both antihistimines and decongestants have been shown to provide relief.

Both dextromethorphan and codeine can depress breathing and should not be used in children under age six to control coughs. They can be used for older children to relieve cough, especially at bedtime. You can continue daily multivitamin pills or drops, but do not dose a child with additional supplements.

Because children tend to get so many colds that last so long, it is often tempting to just try antibiotics, even though we know they're ineffective against viruses. It's just not a good idea. Antibiotics should be used only if there are clear signs of a bacterial infection, such as high fever that develops during the cold and increasing cough and thickened, cloudy mucus. Unnecessary antibiotics can lead to the development of resistant bacteria. Then, when a bacterial infection does occur, the antibiotics may no longer be effective.

Children tend to lose their appetite with a cold. Make sure that they get adequate fluids from tea, water, juice, Jell-O, applesauce, and sherbet. Watch their calorie intake, and if they seem to be taking in few calories, you can entice them with crackers or cookies that are usually not part of their meal plan.

Room air humidifiers can be helpful when your child has a cold and the air is very cold and dry. The extra moisture in the environment helps relieve congestion and decreases risk of bacterial infections. Be careful to change the water every day and clean thoroughly to prevent development of mold, which would then be aerosolized around your home. Follow directions for use on page 50.

SINUSITIS IN CHILDHOOD

While up to 80 percent of adults with colds develop some degree of sinusitis, this occurs far less commonly in children. In fact, only 5–10 percent of children with colds develop problems in the sinus cavities. Unfortunately, when your child's sinuses do become involved, the condition can be difficult to diagnose and to treat. Sinusitis can take several forms. Acute sinusitis is likely when a cold lasts longer than fourteen days but less than thirty days. Chronic sinusitis is suspected when congestion, swelling, and discomfort last more than four weeks. Allergic sinusitis can become better or get worse, but never really goes away. This form of sinusitis is common in families with a history of allergies or eczema. Children who are in day care, have several brothers and sisters, or have parents who smoke in the home may be more likely to develop sinus prob-lems.

Symptoms of Sinusitis in Childhood

In children, it is not so much the severity of the sinus symptoms that causes problems as it is their persistence. Unlike in adults, there is no fever or pain. Children may have bad breath, con-gestion during the day, and a cough at night. It can be difficult to diagnose sinusitis in youngsters. Transillumination (the shin-ing of bright light on the inner rim of the eye socket will light up a healthy sinus, but the congested sinus will remain dark) and CT scans, which are so effective in adults, are less helpful identifying inflamed sinus passages in youngsters. Your child's pediatrician will determine the status of your child's sinuses primarily by observation.

Transmission of Sinusitis in Childhood

In addition to colds and flu, acute sinusitis can develop from other childhood illnesses, such as mumps and measles. Allergies can lead to chronic sinusitis with occasional episodes of acute bacterial flare-ups.

Treatment Issues of Sinusitis in Childhood

Acetaminophen and ibuprofen formulated specifically for chil-dren can be given to reduce discomfort or fever of acute sinusi-tis. When allergies are driving the sinus problems, steroid nasal sprays such as Fluticasone can reduce congestion and inflamma-tion. Antihistamines can be helpful to dry out airways if aller-gies are present. The newer, nonsedating antihistamines are effective, albeit more expensive. The older, less costly, traditional antihistamines can be used effectively at bedtime. Decongestants can be especially helpful. Not only do they open nasal passages, but they also allow steroids to reach affected areas and thus work more efficiently.

When it is clear that your child has acute bacterial sinusitis, a ten-day course of antibiotics is the mainstay of treatment. Amoxicillin is prescribed for most young patients. If there is no improvement within forty-eight hours, it is often wise to change to another class of antibiotics, such as cephalosporins.

Water in different forms is a troubled sinus's best friend. Ice packs on the eye areas can relieve pain and a sense of congestion. Saline drops in the nose will loosen dry, hardened mucus in babies and toddlers. Older children can use nasal syringes with a bulb or nebulizer. Youngsters old enough to shower by themselves will find the moist, warm atmosphere helps them to breathe. Warm soup and tea are also beneficial to relieve congestion, so be sure to provide fluids.

Traditional sinus surgery is not recommended for children under age five. New types of endoscopic surgery remove obstructions at the point where the mucus flows from all three sinuses converge. The result is significantly better drainage with less invasive surgery. Any type of surgery is usually reserved for children who have not responded to all other medical options.

BRONCHITIS IN CHILDHOOD

While bronchitis is a frequent fellow traveler with colds and flu in adults, it is far more unusual in children. Youngsters who live in homes where parents are smokers or those who have allergies are at higher risk to develop bronchitis after a viral infection.

Symptoms of Bronchitis in Childhood

Bronchitis in children starts with a dry cough that soon becomes thick with mucus. Fever is usually absent and the child does not feel or seem to be ill. Symptoms disappear within seven to ten days.

Treatment of Bronchitis in Childhood

Bronchitis usually gets better by itself. If the cough is troubling, start off treating with a lozenge or cough drop. Hot tea with honey and lemon will provide soothing moisture. In most cases, childhood bronchitis is an irritation reaction rather than a secondary bacterial infection, so antibiotics are generally not needed. If a cough persists, call your child's pediatrician to determine the cause.

STREP THROAT IN CHILDHOOD

While sinusitis and bronchitis are not usual childhood illnesses, strep throat is all too common. Each year, more than 7 million youngsters are treated for strep. Before World War II, strep outbreaks occurred in distinct clusters. Since the 1940s, strep is common all year round, with peak incidence in winter and early spring.

Symptoms of Strep in Childhood

Strep throat arrives suddenly and dramatically, with sore throat and fever. Headaches, nausea, vomiting, and stomach pain are frequently seen. Tonsils are enlarged, neck glands are swollen, and even the tongue can be red and puffy. However, if symptoms include a cough or congestion in the nose, the cause is likely to be a cold or flu virus, rather than strep bacteria.

Complications of Strep in Childhood

Up to 25 percent of strep throats fail to respond completely, even after complete antibiotic treatment. Pain, fever, and other symptoms are gone, but the throat cultures are still positive for the bacteria. Called *carriage,* it can spread infection to others or may flare up again in your child. While it does not increase the risk of rheumatic fever, carriage of strep requires prompt treatments with antibiotics at the first sign of new symptoms. Carriage can last six to twelve months and require vigilance by parents and doctors.

Concerns about strep recurrence are due to a now uncommon complication of strep infection—rheumatic fever. For reasons that we still don't fully understand, the streptococcus bacteria provokes intense inflammation throughout the body. In the joints it causes swelling and pain. When the inflammation reaches the heart, it can cause permanent scarring of the myocardium, the lining of the heart. Although the incidence of rheumatic fever is sharply reduced, your pediatrician will be watchful that your child's strep infections are completely resolved.

Treatment Issues of Strep in Childhood

Penicillin, four times a day for ten days, is still the gold standard for treating strep throat. More recently, amoxicillin has been prescribed for ten days. It can be moderately difficult to convince a child over five to take antibiotic emulsions or pills. When it comes to a balky baby or toddler, it can be impossible. To ensure adequate treatment, your pediatrician may choose a one-dose injection of penicillin. If your child has a penicillin allergy, erythromycin emulsion or pills, two to three times a day for ten days, can bring the strep infection under control.

Until the 1970s, tonsils and adenoids were routinely removed if a child had several episodes of strep throat. By the

1980s, doctors realized that the risks of surgery outweighed the reduction in number of infections. Tonsillectomies are now reserved only for cases where tonsils are so enlarged that they interfere with swallowing. Adenoids are removed only when obstruction is so severe it makes breathing difficult, or when chronic ear infections do not respond to medical treatment.

PNEUMONIA IN CHILDHOOD

Pneumonia is usually viewed as a disease of older people, but it can affect children of all ages. For infants less than four months, pneumonia usually requires hospitalization for treatment. The three general types of pneumonia—viral, bacterial, and mycoplasmal—tend to affect different age groups of children.

Viral Pneumonia

Viruses are the most common cause of pneumonia in children ages four months to four years. Viral pneumonia starts suddenly with wheezing, shortness of breath, and nasal congestion. In small children, there are often GI problems such as diarrhea and nausea. On X-ray, doctors can see the lungs are overexpanded. Much of viral pneumonia is associated with influenza. Adenovirus and parainfluenza virus, which cause colds in adults, can also produce pneumonia in children. About 25 percent of viral pneumonia in children under age two is due to respiratory syncytial virus, also known as RSV.

Viral pneumonia in infants is always serious and usually requires hospitalization. Breathing is carefully monitored and oxygen support is often required. Treatment is focused on providing support until the body can overcome the viral infection. If doctors are concerned that a bacterial infection may be developing in the congested lungs, antibiotics may be prescribed. The single best way to prevent viral pneumonia is to ensure that your child is vaccinated each year against influenza. Although other viruses may cause pneumonia in children, the most serious and the most common are the result of the influenza virus. Vaccination can have a major impact in reducing your child's risk of developing viral pneumonia. Current CDC guidelines recommend that all babies between the ages of six and twenty-three months receive the flu shot. Further down the list, the CDC recommendations include the shot for all persons over the age of six months who "wish to reduce the likelihood of becoming ill with the flu."

Bacterial Pneumonia

It is estimated that 10 percent of all pneumonia in children is caused by bacteria. Newborns and children with underlying health problems such as asthma or cystic fibrosis are at higher risk for bacterial pneumonia. Babies less than one month old will usually need to be hospitalized. The most likely cause is *Streptococcus pneumoniae,* an organism in the same family of bacteria that cause strep throat. *Haemophilus influenzae,* another bacterium, is less common, but certainly a suspect.

Bacterial pneumonia often starts with coldlike symptoms, including fever, cough, earache, and congestion. Within a day, breathing rate increases, skin may take on a bluish tone, and children complain of chest pain. Babies and toddlers seem to struggle to breathe with flaring nostrils and grunting sounds. Bacterial pneumonia can last a week to ten days, but the child may feel listless and unable to return to school for several weeks thereafter. Pulmonary function may be weakened for months, and children will tire more easily.

Until recently, the pneumonia vaccine used for adults did not work well for young children. Now a new "conjugate" vaccine, which uses a dead bacteria, is extremely effective even for children under age two. It provides immunity against the seven most common strains of pneumococcus that cause serious infection in children. Infants get four doses, one each at two, four, six, and twelve to fifteen months. Children who begin the series later will not need all four doses. Youngsters over age five will generally not need the conjugate vaccine. Older children who have underlying health problems may be given one or both of the vaccines; that is, both the vaccine for children and that for adults. Side effects of the pneumococcal vaccine are generally limited to a bit of redness at the injection site or fever. If a child has a severe reaction to one shot in the series, the other injections may be suspended. A shot should also be postponed if a child has a moderate to severe illness at the time the shot is scheduled.

The choice of antibiotics to treat bacterial pneumonia depends on the age of the child and the bacteria causing the illness. Infants three weeks to three months of age respond well to erythromycin. Between four months and four years, amoxicillin is the antibiotic of choice. From five to fifteen years, erythromycin again seems to be the most desirable antibiotic.

Mycoplasma Pneumonia

Mycoplasma are a form of bacteria that are larger than viruses, but much smaller than most bacterial organisms. Although little known, they are actually the leading cause of pneumonia in children ages five to fifteen. It is also the only form of pneumonia that is truly contagious and can be spread from person to person. The rate of contagion is slow, so it can spread for months in a family or a school. It is common in communities where children live closely together, such as dormitories, camps, and institutions.

Mycoplasma pneumonia initially appears like an ordinary cold, with symptoms of fever, sore throat, and cough. The symptoms are mild, but when a doctor listens to a child's chest, he can hear rales and rhonchi, chest sounds that are much more severe than would be expected from the mild respiratory symptoms. If properly treated, mycoplasma pneumonia will persist for about fourteen days. But treatment is often delayed because the parents and physicians are unaware that the problem is ongoing. A child can feel tired and have a cough for weeks before it is properly diagnosed. Basic hygiene precautions can limit its spread in a community. Hand washing and covering nose and mouth when sneezing and coughing are believed to reduce the spread of infection.

The macrolide antibiotics, such as erythromycin, have been proven effective for mycoplasma pneumonia. A seven-to-ten-day course of erythromycin is usually the treatment of choice. Interestingly, mycoplasmas are resistant to penicillin and cephalosporins, because these organisms lack the cell walls that are susceptible to these antibiotics. In fact, the first sign that a physician may be looking at a mycoplasma pneumonia infection often comes when a respiratory infection fails to respond to penicillin or cephalosporin. Tetracycline is another antibiotic option prescribed for children eight years old and up.

INFLUENZA

Influenza hits children hard. In a flu outbreak, about 20 percent of adults come down with symptoms. By contrast, over half of children in a community will develop influenza during the flu season. In children younger than six months, the symptoms can be particularly severe and the mortality rate can equal that of elderly people with underlying health problems. In addition to traditional flu symptoms of cough, fever, and body aches, children can get conjunctivitis and GI symptoms, such as nausea, vomiting, or stomach pains. Ear infections are also common and develop about 50 percent of the time in children with flu. Hospitalization rates for children less than two years old are twelve times that for older children.

Never use aspirin in treating children with congestion and

fever because of the risk of Reye's syndrome (see page 177). Because high fevers can provoke seizures in children, it is important to control this symptom with acetaminophen or ibuprofen. The dosage of these anti-inflammatory agents is based on age and body weight. Read the manufacturer's product labeling carefully to determine how much of and how often these should be given to your child and never exceed the recommended dosage. To keep track, keep a small notebook to record at what time and how much of these agents were given. This is a useful tool in recapping your treatments when consulting your child's pediatrician.

For children with underlying health problems, such as asthma, cystic fibrosis, or sickle-cell anemia, doctors can recommend antiviral agents such as Tamiflu to be given in the first forty-eight hours of influenza infection. In families with a large number of children or that also care for an elderly relative, antiviral agents also help control the shedding of virus and thus limit the spread of influenza.

There are a range of flu vaccine options for every age to prevent this infection every year. Some parents have expressed concerns about a preservative that is used in vaccines called thimerosal and its possible link to the development of autism. While most studies do not indicate a link, if you are concerned about thimerosal, try the new flu vaccine Fluvirin, which is prepared with an alternative preservative.

Two major forms of vaccine are available for healthy children: the injectable vaccine and an inhaled vaccine. The injectable vaccine is made from conjugate, or dead viruses. Like the adult vaccine, it contains three strains; however, it is prepared from a split product that produces fewer reactions than the adult vaccine would in children. The amount of vaccine is also dependent on the age of the child, with smaller amounts of vaccine given in one to two doses in children ages six months to eight years. In addition, from nine to twelve years, a single dose is given.

For healthy children from five to eighteen years, the inhaled flu vaccine FluMist can provide a safe, effective, and needle-free vaccination. This type of vaccine uses an inactivated virus that is not recommended for children with underlying health problems. In children younger than nine years old, two doses are given, separated by six to ten weeks. This vaccine can be given the same day as the measles, mumps, rubella, or chicken pox vaccination. If it is not given on the same day, then the flu vaccine should be given no earlier than four weeks later. Interestingly, flu vaccines also seem to decrease the incidence of ear infections. About 2 percent of children under twelve have some fever after vaccination.

There are two levels of recommendations for flu vaccines. Absolute indications mean that the vaccine should be standard in any healthy-baby program. In addition, recommendation guidelines mean that the vaccine can be an option at the discretion of both the parents and the pediatrician. Current guidelines recommend that all children ages six to twenty-three months receive the vaccine. It is suggested that children older than two who want to avoid the flu should also receive it. Children under the age of nine who are receiving flu vaccine for their first time should get it split into two doses, separated by one month. For the live, inactivated vaccine that is the inhaled form, children five to eight years old should receive two doses separated by six to ten weeks. To protect both your child and family, I recommend flu vaccinations for children of all ages.

Antibiotics should only be used if your child's pediatrician knows or strongly suspects that there is a bacterial superinfection, such as bronchitis or pneumonia. Antibiotics will not prevent viral infections, and needless use can only increase risk of resistance, which means that when they are truly needed to fight an infection, they may not be effective.

BRONCHIOLITIS

In addition to the standard six respiratory infections that affect adults and children, children have three infections of their very own: bronchiolitis, croup, and otitis media, also known as ear-ache. Bronchiolitis is the most common, serious, acute respiratory illness in infants and young children. It occurs in epidemics in distinct seasonal patterns. In temperate climates, such as that of the United States, it begins in winter and ends in early spring. In tropical climates, bronchiolitis occurs in the rainy season. It is spread by contact, so frequent and thorough hand washing is our best defense.

Bronchiolitis begins with typical cold symptoms. After one or two days, wheezing develops. Your child looks and feels acutely ill. Breathing is shallow and rapid, while X-rays will show mildly inflated lungs. Most children start to show improvement within three to four days, with gradual recovery in one to two weeks. A severe attack of bronchiolitis in childhood seems to significantly increase the child's risk of developing asthma.

Causes of Bronchiolitis

Up to 75 percent of bronchiolitis is caused by the respiratory syncytial virus, known as RSV. Biologically, RSV is related to the pneumovirus. By age one, 50 percent of all children have had some type of RSV infection. By age three, that number has risen to 100 percent. Unfortunately, infection with RSV does not develop immunity to future RSV illness. In most cases, the RSV illness is mild and written off as a standard cold. But RSV is not always such an invisible enemy. Each year, eighty thousand children are hospitalized with severe RSV infections such as bronchiolitis.

Bronchiolitis is more common in children with underlying health problems, such as cystic fibrosis, heart disease, asthma, and even premature birth. Other factors that increase the chance of developing severe bronchiolitis include a history of allergy in the family, very young mothers, pollution, and large numbers of brothers and sisters.

Treatment Issues of Bronchiolitis

There are a range of opinions on how best to manage bronchiolitis. Some studies indicate that inhaled corticosteroids can reduce virus-induced inflammation of the airways. Other research does not show the same benefits.

Ribavirin is an antiviral agent that has been shown to reduce viral replication. Although clinical trials have not shown widespread success, ribavirin is often given to children with bronchiolitis who also suffer from underlying health problems.

Bronchodilators that are used for asthma management have been shown to keep airways open during an episode of bronchiolitis. They are frequently combined with corticosteroids, and the benefits are greater than when either is used alone.

Prevention of Bronchiolitis

Attempts to make a commercial RSV vaccine have not been successful. An RSV vaccine used in the 1960s actually increased severity of the bronchiolitis symptoms. Currently pediatricians can offer infants at high risk of RSV infections a series of monthly antibody injections. They have been shown to be effective for premature infants as well as children under two with chronic lung disease. The treatment is expensive and is not safe for children with congenital heart disease, but in the right situations, the treatment can be a lifesaver.

OTITIS MEDIA (EARACHE)

Otitis media is an infection caused by the collection of fluid behind the ear drum in the middle ear. For children under fifteen, it is the most frequent diagnosis. The peak incidence is from six to twenty-four months. By their third birthday, two-thirds of children have had at least one episode.

Symptoms of Otitis Media

It starts with fever and pain. Children seem irritable, congested, and lose their appetite. Your child's pediatrician will be able to see that the tympanic membrane in the ear is swollen and inflamed. Fluid persists in the ear long after the active infection is gone. In fact, 70 percent of children have fluid in the ear two weeks after all other symptoms have disappeared.

Causes of Otitis Media

Otitis media is almost always part of a respiratory infection. It can occur as part of a routine cold or flu. Sometimes it can be caused by *Streptococcus pneumoniae* in children who have not received the pneumonia vaccine. Occasionally it can be from an *H. influenzae* infection. While the most common strain of this bacterium is controlled by a vaccine, the type of *H. influenzae* that causes earaches is not covered by the vaccine. Children who are in day care, who drink their bottle lying down, or who are exposed to cigarette smoke in their home are at higher risk for developing otitis media.

Transmission of Otitis Media

The organisms that cause this common infection are both airborne and spread by contact. Under normal circumstances, the middle ear drains by a short, narrow tube (called the eustachian) into the nasal passages. During a cold or flu, the increased congestion blocks the drainage. The eustachian tube becomes closed off and swells with fluid. This built-up fluid becomes infected with bacteria. Children are more vulnerable because their eustachian tube is level to the nasal passages. As we grow older and our face lengthens, the eustachian tubes angle downward, increasing drainage.

Diagnosis of Otitis Media

Diagnosis is made by looking into the ear using an *otoscope,* an instrument with a bright light that allows the doctor to see the eardrum. Normally the eardrum membrane is flat and pink. In an ear infection, the membrane is swollen, bulging outward, and yellow or red.

Complications of Otitis Media

Some degree of temporary hearing loss may linger for months after an ear infection. In children with repeated episodes of otitis media, the hearing loss may be permanent. Studies indicate that these children may show delays in language development and lower test scores in speech and reasoning.

Prevention of Otitis Media

While it is impossible to avoid all respiratory infections, steps can be taken to lower the risk of developing otitis media. The annual flu shot will prevent ear infections associated with influenza. Feed your baby his or her bottles in a semi-upright position. Keeping your home tobacco-free has been shown to lower incidence of otitis media in children of all ages.

The vaccine for pneumonia has been shown to cut the incidence of ear infections. For children with a history of frequent ear infections, some doctors recommend a six-week course of antibiotics during the height of the cold and flu season, but this approach is controversial.

Treatment Issues of Otitis Media

Acetaminophen or ibuprofen formulated for children can be given to reduce pain and fever. Antihistamines have been shown to be effective where allergies may be increasing fluid buildup. Decongestants are often prescribed, but their effectiveness is debated.

Antibiotics are usually prescribed for ten days to completely knock out otitis media. Amoxicillin is the most frequently prescribed antibiotic, closely followed by Ceftin. If the pain and fever are not gone in two days, call your physician to discuss the need for another antibiotic. The antibiotic may not be effective against the type of bacteria that is causing the infection, or the bacteria may have developed resistance to the antibiotics. Recently, there has been a trend to limit antibiotics to severe ear infections.

CROUP

Croup is an obstruction of the upper airways in young children. It primarily affects children ages six months to three years and seems to strike more boys than girls. Epidemics of croup begin in the fall and peak in early winter. Children who get an episode of croup have an increased risk for developing asthma.

Symptoms of Croup

One to two days after the start of a cold or flu, the onset of croup is sudden and unexpected. Your child develops a barking cough and strains to breathe. Other signs include laryngitis, a hoarse cry, or a wheezing sound when the child inhales. Episodes often start after a child has been asleep for several hours. In 90 percent of cases, the symptoms are mild and manageable at home. Those with moderate or severe croup may wind up in the ER.

Causes of Croup

Both viruses and bacteria can trigger croup. The annual influenza virus is a common cause of croup. In addition, the parainfluenza and adenoviruses that cause typical colds in adults are among the leading croup-producing organisms.

Until 1985, *Haemophilus influenzae,* a common bacterium, was the single leading cause of croup. Known as Hib, it struck one child in two hundred under the age of five. Each year eight thousand children died from Hib-induced bronchospasm. With the introduction of a safe, effective vaccine, Hib-induced croup has practically disappeared in Western countries.

Today Hib vaccines are made by several different manufacturers. Children get three to four doses, depending on the brand of vaccine. All children should get the vaccine at two and four months and a booster between twelve and fifteen months. It can also be combined in the same shot as the DPT or hepatitis B. If your child is older than age five, there is no need for an Hib immunization.

Treatment of Croup

The age-old therapy for croup is steam. In the past century parents held their croupy child over a steaming teakettle. To avoid the risk of scalding your child with hot water, take your child into the bathroom and run a hot shower to fill the room with clouds of steam. *Do not put the child in the hot shower or bath.* Hold your child in your arms and allow the steam to work. Relief should occur in ten minutes. If the child is not breathing easily in twenty minutes, call your doctor or go to the local Emergency Department immediately.

By the time you arrive at the Emergency Department, you may be surprised to find that your little one may be breathing comfortably. Paradoxically, cold, dry night air has also been shown to relieve croup. Doctors believe that the cold air shrinks swollen blood vessels, thus reducing obstruction in the airways.

If breathing continues to be labored, doctors may use a combination of inhaled epinephrine and corticosteroids. Because relief may only be temporary, your child may stay in the Emergency Department for several hours to be watched for new signs of airway spasm. Croup usually lasts three to four days. During this time your child will feel better during the day, but symptoms may return at night. Antibiotics are not prescribed if the cause is viral, but may be given if doctors suspect a bacterial infection has developed.

Prevention of Croup

Three vaccines have dramatically cut the number of children who develop croup symptoms. The annual flu shot plus the pneumonia and Hib vaccines have changed the severity and incidence of childhood respiratory infections. I believe that they are among the major advances in health care in the last twenty-five years and should be part of well-baby care for all children.

CHAPTER 11

Individual Needs, Individual Solutions

ONE SIZE DOES NOT FIT ALL

Individual health issues such as pregnancy change the dynamics of colds and flu in different ways. Some problems such as diabetes can increase the susceptibility to catching a respiratory infection. Other situations call for changes in the way we handle symptoms. For example, many people with asthma have an allergy to aspirin and should choose acetaminophen to relieve fever and body aches.

This chapter examines three issues: (1) how an underlying medical issue affects the development of a cold or flu; (2) how a respiratory infection affects the underlying health issue; and (3) what changes are needed in the standard treatment plan. This chapter will look at six of the most common situations—asthma, diabetes, hypertension, COPD, pregnancy, and health issues of seniors. Each section begins with a brief overview of the disease or health issue and a discussion of its impact on colds and flu. It closes with a review of the standard treatment components and how and why adjustments should be made.

WHEN PREVENTION GOES TOO FAR

In the fall of 2004, the shortage of flu shots led to earnest advice on the value of taking preventive measures. There were recommendations for washing hands at least twenty seconds, ten times a day, wearing gloves when dealing with people, and strapping on a face mask when going outside. At some point the advice crossed the line from generally accepted guidelines into obsessive-compulsive behavior.

I want you to be aware of ways that you can lessen your exposure to illness-causing organisms, but not at the price of altering the quality of your life. Use preventive measures sensibly. If you work with someone who clearly has a cold, don't borrow his pen, shake hands, or use his phone. But don't be afraid of being with your family and friends. Go to movies, restaurants, and parties. Enjoy your life without the fear that germs are lurking on every surface. If you do catch a cold or flu, well, that's what this book is for.

ASTHMA

Asthma is a chronic inflammatory disorder of the airways caused by our reactions to allergens and irritants. When our airways come into contact with these triggers, they respond with a cascade of changes that leads to narrowing of the airways, swelling of the bronchial tissues, and production of thick mucus. This results in feelings of chest tightness, coughing, and difficulty in breathing.

A wide range of medications can help keep airways open, reduce inflammation, and prevent full-blown asthmatic attacks. However, the already-inflamed asthmatic airways are particularly vulnerable to the effects of a respiratory infection. If you have asthma, there is no such thing as a little cold. Asthmatic airways are more susceptible to the viruses in the environment.

Not only are infections more frequent, complications such as bronchitis and pneumonia are generally more common. Even a simple respiratory infection tends to be more severe and long-lasting and may provoke an acute asthmatic episode. Over time, a combination of drawn-out colds and asthmatic attacks can lead to permanent obstruction in the airways that cannot be reversed with medications.

To prevent these problems, colds and other respiratory infections need to be taken seriously from the first sniffle. I ask my patients to call me when they start to feel the first symptoms of a cold so we can be on the lookout for indications that the asthma is worsening and additional airway medication may be needed.

Treatment Issues of Asthma and Respiratory Infections

ANTI-INFLAMMATORY DRUGS. Asthmatics need to avoid aspirin. About 10 percent of asthmatics are allergic to aspirin, and a single dose can trigger wheezing. In some cases, an asthmatic can be allergic to all types of medication classified as nonsteroidal anti-inflammatory drugs (NSAIDs), including ibuprofen and Anaprox. To safely reduce the discomfort of colds and flu in people with asthma, I recommend the use of acetaminophen (Tylenol).

ANTIHISTAMINES. Since asthma is often caused by allergies, antihistamines are effective in reducing the production of mucus-producing histamine. They are especially helpful in children, in whom 90 percent of asthma is due to allergies.

DECONGESTANTS. Several of the medications used to keep airways open and comfortable tend to increase heart rate and blood pressure. Since decongestants can also have this effect, it would be wise to limit their use.

VACCINES. Asthmatics are included in the high-risk category for influenza and are in the first groups of persons who should receive the flu vaccine. Studies confirm that influenza vaccination is safe and effective if you have asthma. Immunization for pneumonia is equally helpful.

ANTIVIRALS. Tamiflu can be extremely helpful for asthmatics who get the flu. Remember, the flu vaccine is 70 to 80 percent effective, so flu may develop despite the shot. You may have received the shot too late to develop antibodies before exposure, or you may have caught a random flu virus that was not included in the vaccine. It is important to note that the other antiviral medication, Relenza, which causes wheezing and shortness of breath in asthmatics, should be avoided.

COUGH CONTROL. Asthma often causes a severe cough, and an additional infection can make a bad situation worse. To provide relief I often prescribe additional bronchodilators as well as cough suppressants that include dextromethorphan or codeine. It is occasionally necessary to use corticosteroid spray for several weeks to break the asthma/cough cycle.

SUPPLEMENTS. Asthmatics can use zinc lozenges and vitamin C (up to 500 mg/day) to treat cold symptoms. For an asthmatic I tend to discourage the use of all herbals including echinacea. These plants may contain pollen and other allergens and may contribute to asthma symptoms.

ANTIBIOTICS. The already damaged and inflamed airways of asthmatics increase susceptibility to secondary bacterial infections. Therefore, for my asthmatic patients I tend to prescribe antibiotics sooner rather than later. Even though antibiotics have no impact on the viruses that cause colds and flu, in chronically inflamed airways bacterial sinusitis and bronchitis can develop quickly.

NUTRITION. Large epidemiological studies have indi-cated that people whose diets are rich in fruits and veg-etables have lower rates of asthma. It is suggested that the high levels of antioxidants in these foods reduce free radicals, which are elevated in the lungs of people with asthma. If you don't feel up to big salads and stir-fried broccoli, you can get a healthy supply of antioxidants from hot soups made with a variety of vegetables. Hot tea with lemon, cold orange juice, and lemonade provide fluids and plenty of vitamin C, a proven free-radical fighter.

HYDROTHERAPY. Hot showers in the morning will pro-vide essential moisture for sensitive asthmatic airways, which are easily dehydrated during a respiratory infection.

DIABETES

Diabetes is a chronic disorder in which the body cannot prop-erly metabolize sugar. Normally the pancreas produces a hor-mone called insulin that helps cells utilize sugar for growth and energy. If the body is unable to produce sufficient insulin or is unable to utilize existing insulin, sugar levels in the blood rise dramatically and dangerously in the body. In the short run, high blood sugar levels can lead to fatal diabetic coma. Over time, even mildly elevated blood sugar levels destroy blood vessels in vital organs. Abnormal blood sugar levels can rupture blood vessels in the eyes, leading to irreversible blindness. Diabetes hardens capillaries of the kidneys, leading to kidney failure. Damaged blood vessels in the heart increase the risk of strokes and heart attacks. Fortunately, studies have shown that by keeping blood sugar levels within a normal range we can cut the rate of these devastating complications by as much as 70 percent.

When managing diabetes, our goal is to use diet, exercise, and medication to help patients keep their blood sugar at healthy levels. Colds and flu can disrupt good diabetic control in two ways. High sugar levels have a devastating effect on our immune system. In fact, one of the key symptoms of undiagnosed diabetes is repeated infections, such as urinary and respiratory infections. This decreased immunity also increases the risk of complications such as bronchitis and pneumonia.

To add further problems, respiratory infections themselves tend to raise blood sugar levels. This increase not only affects good sugar control in diabetes, it further weakens the ability to deal with an infection. To avoid this downward spiral, you and your physician need to aggressively treat respiratory infections as well as closely monitor blood sugar levels. You will need to test your blood sugar more often, and if the numbers are running higher than normal, discuss treatment options with your physician. If you are on oral medications, you may need to increase the dosage or add a new category of drug to control blood sugar levels during the illness. If you are on insulin, the doctor may increase units or change to a longer-lasting form to provide better coverage. If you are too sick to eat, use nondiet soft drinks for both calories and fluids.

HEALTH ALERT FOR DIABETICS

If you are taking metformin (Glucophage) and have a fever over 102, vomiting, or feel short of breath, stop taking metformin immediately and call your physician. In acute illness, metformin can lead to a life-threatening problem known as lactic acidosis.

Treatment Issues of Diabetes and Respiratory Infections

ANTI-INFLAMMATORY. Diabetics can safely use aspirin, acetaminophen, and ibuprofen. Use them early and often to control symptoms. Fever tends to raise blood sugar, and these inexpensive over-the-counter aids will keep fever under control.

ANTIHISTAMINES. These are helpful for reducing sneezing and congestion. Be sure to take them in pill or capsule form because most of the liquid and syrup products are high in sugar.

DECONGESTANTS. While they can provide genuine relief for cold symptoms, decongestants have been known to raise blood sugar levels in people with diabetes. Test their impact by measuring blood sugar levels before and after decongestant use. If your blood sugar remains well controlled, they can be used in small doses. If the blood sugar numbers rise, avoid them entirely.

VACCINES. A yearly flu shot is essential. The vaccine for pneumonia should be repeated every ten years for full coverage.

ANTIVIRALS. Tamiflu and Relenza are often prescribed when people with diabetes come down with the flu. Since they need to be taken in the first forty-eight hours of infection, physicians often recommend that a course of one of these drugs be on hand in your medicine chest to use at the first sign of flu symptoms.

COUGH CONTROL. Try to avoid traditional cough drops, cough syrups, and liquid cold medicines since they are often high in sugar. Use capsules and pills or look for sugar-free cough syrups. If a physician prescribes a codeine cough syrup, diabetics should ask their pharmacist for a sugar-free formula.

SUPPLEMENTS. Look for sugar-free zinc lozenges or use the nasal swabs or spray. Vitamin C supplements are important since orange juice is high in sugar and not recommended in a diabetic food plan.

ANTIBIOTICS. Since diabetics are more susceptible to bacterial infections, the threshold for use is lower. If cold symptoms do not improve within three days, or the cough seems to be getting worse, antibiotics may be needed. Avoid a quinolone antibiotic called Tequin, which has been found to raise blood sugar levels in diabetics.

NUTRITION. Watch the sugar content of foods consumed during a respiratory illness. Avoid fruit juices and select no-sugar-added ice cream, puddings, and Jell-O. Use non-caloric sweeteners with your hot tea and lemon. When we feel feverish and achy, we tend to gravitate to easy-to-digest carbohydrates such as toast, cake, and cookies. These foods should always be eaten in small quantities by people with diabetes, and carb loading during a respiratory illness will probably make you feel worse.

PREGNANCY

When a cold or flu strikes during pregnancy, two questions arise: How will the infection affect the pregnant woman, and what is the impact on the baby? The primary goal, of course, is to make sure that the health and well-being of both are protected. While we certainly need to treat the respiratory infection, we need to ensure that the medications do not cause problems for the developing fetus.

The first step is to prevent as many infections as possible.

Frequent hand washing cuts down on transmission of colds and strep throats. In flu season I recommend avoiding crowds during pregnancy. However, if this is not your first pregnancy, your own children will likely bring home viruses and it will be necessary to treat them in a way that protects the health of both you and your baby.

Although most infections are uncomfortable, they do not pose a health threat for an otherwise healthy mother. However, influenza can be serious to both mother and child. Influenza during pregnancy can lead to complications such as miscarriage and stillbirth. Babies whose mothers had contracted the flu during pregnancy have been reported to be at increased risk for developing schizophrenia in later life. The risks of flu during pregnancy are so significant that both the Centers for Disease Control and Prevention (CDC) and the Advisory Committee on Immunization Practices (ACIP) recommend getting the influenza vaccine at any point in pregnancy.

Pregnancy can increase the discomfort of even a mild cold. Due to increased fluid levels in pregnancy, many women feel chronically congested. When a cold strikes, the additional swelling in the airways can make you feel as if you were trying to breathe underwater.

Treatment Issues of Pregnancy and Respiratory Infections

ANTI-INFLAMMATORY. Acetaminophen (e.g., Tylenol) is probably the most important tool to provide relief for respiratory infections during pregnancy. However, it is important not to exceed recommended dosage to avoid potential liver problems. Aspirin has been shown to cause congenital birth defects and should be avoided. Ibuprofen has been linked to a serious lung disorder in the baby called pulmonary hypertension, and many physicians caution against its use in pregnant women.

ANTIHISTAMINES. These are not recommended during pregnancy. Some studies indicate a rise in the risk of birth defects from the use of several widely used antihistamines. These findings have led to recommendations to avoid all forms of this medication while pregnant.

DECONGESTANTS. Blood pressure can become elevated during pregnancy. Since decongestants themselves can raise blood pressure, doctors tend to caution against their use in pregnancy.

VACCINES. The flu shot is important for pregnant women. Because influenza in the mother can increase the risk of miscarriage and stillbirth, all the major health associations recommend the fall/winter influenza shot at whatever time in the pregnancy that season occurs.

ANTIVIRALS. Despite the dangers of the flu to mother and baby, these medications cannot be used during pregnancy. Reports indicate a small increased risk of birth defects with their use, and doctors feel that the risks of the treatment outweigh the benefits of the drugs.

COUGH CONTROL. Avoid all liquid cough preparations because they are 20 percent ethanol (alcohol), which is known to cause birth defects. Never use codeine-based cough products, since this narcotic can depress the baby's central nervous system. Try to control the cough with sugar- or honey-based lozenges. If more cough control is needed, look for pills or lozenges that contain dextromethorphan if you are bringing up mucus, or guaifenesin if the cough is dry and hard.

SUPPLEMENTS. Except for a daily prenatal multivitamin, taking supplements is not a good idea during pregnancy. Many vitamins, including A and D in high doses, have been shown to cause birth defects. Infants whose mothers consumed large amounts of vitamin C supplements developed scurvy soon after birth. Avoid all herbs, including echinacia, whose safety has not been demonstrated.

ANTIBIOTICS. Birth defects have been identified for a number of usually safe and well-tolerated antibiotics. Tetracycline has been shown to cause tooth discoloration and inhibition of bone growth if used during the last six months of pregnancy. Quinolones should be avoided because they have been associated with the development of joint problems in children whose mothers took these drugs during pregnancy. If an antibiotic is needed to combat a bacterial infection, penicillin, erythromycin, and clindamycins are usually considered safe and effective for both mother and unborn baby.

NUTRITION. During pregnancy the diet needs to nourish both mother and child. Although you may lose your appetite with a respiratory illness, try to take in adequate calories and nutrients, and keep in mind that fluid needs, which are already increased during pregnancy, are further increased with a fever. Be sure to avoid salt in your food and use low-sodium chicken soups for cold and flu relief.

HYDROTHERAPY. Given that antihistamines, decongestants, and antivirals cannot be used during pregnancy, water in different forms becomes increasingly important to relieve discomfort. Be sure to drink two to three cups of decaffeinated hot tea, as well as three to four glasses of cold water with a slice of lime or lemon, to provide adequate hydration. Use a saline nasal rinse to relieve congestion and a saline gargle to soothe a sore throat. A warm shower in the morning will help you breathe easier during the day.

CHRONIC OBSTRUCTIVE PULMONARY DISEASE (COPD)

COPD is an umbrella term for a group of related diseases including chronic bronchitis and emphysema. Although it is the fourth leading cause of death in the United States, only half of the estimated 26 million Americans affected are aware that their shortness of breath and lingering cough are signs of a serious illness.

COPD results from long-term irritation to the airways such as from cigarette smoke and workplace pollution. The constant irritation provokes excess mucus production, which over time blocks the airways. The lining of the airways becomes thickened and inflamed, making it hard to breathe. In emphysema the inflammation actually destroys the alveoli, the tiny grapelike structures where oxygen is exchanged for carbon dioxide, and thus the very basis for breathing. It is no wonder, then, that the key symptom of COPD is chronic shortness of breath.

In COPD the airways are frequently filled with excess mucus that can trigger a constant cough. This mucus accumulation is an ideal place for bacteria to grow. When a cold or flu virus infects the airways in a person with COPD, the additional inflammation can quickly lead to bronchitis or pneumonia. In addition, people with COPD can develop what is called an acute exacerbation. Symptoms of an acute exacerbation include fever, increasing shortness of breath, and a worsening, phlegm-laden cough. This serious illness is the leading cause of hospitalization for people with COPD. Many need to be admitted to the intensive care unit to provide careful monitoring of their vital signs. Even with all the best resources, mortality of COPD in an intensive care unit approaches 50 percent. In those who do recover, there is often a permanent decline in lung function. They will have more shortness of breath and need more and/or additional medications. Not infrequently, after a difficult exacerbation, they will need to use oxygen twenty-four hours a day.

To prevent problems before they start, my COPD patients know that I need to hear from them at the first sign of a sniffle or fever. The earlier we can work to control the respiratory infection, the better the outcome.

Treatment Issues of COPD and Respiratory Infections

ANTI-INFLAMMATORY. I recommend using acetaminophen (Tylenol) or ibuprofen (Motrin) rather than aspirin. Many people with COPD also have asthma, and about 10 percent of people with asthma are allergic to aspirin.

ANTIHISTAMINES. Both traditional sedating and newer nonsedating antihistamines can be used safely and effectively.

DECONGESTANTS. Some of the medications prescribed for COPD tend to raise heart rate. In addition, most people with COPD are at an age where high blood pressure is common. Because decongestants can also increase blood pressure, they should be used with caution in people with COPD.

VACCINES. All people with COPD are at the top of the list for yearly flu vaccinations. The pneumonia vaccine is equally important and should be repeated every ten years.

ANTIVIRALS. If influenza does strike, the antiviral Tamiflu is an excellent option if taken in the first forty-eight hours after symptoms began.

SUPPLEMENTS. Studies have shown that people whose diets are high in antioxidants have a lower risk of developing COPD, even in those who smoked cigarettes. Unfortunately, supplements of antioxidants such as vitamin A, beta-carotene, and vitamin E do not provide the same pulmonary-protective benefits. COPD patients can use zinc and up to five hundred milligrams daily of vitamin C to reduce cold symptoms.

ANTIBIOTICS. While antibiotics have no benefits against routine viral colds and flu, when COPD is present, the threshold for prescribing antibiotics is much lower. Because secondary bacterial infections can happen so quickly, I give my COPD patients a prescription for antibiotics to have on hand if a respiratory infection develops. They know to call me before starting any medication, but it's reassuring to both of us that the antibiotics are at hand to avert an acute exacerbation.

HYPERTENSION

High blood pressure or hypertension is a common disorder in which the pressure in the arteries is too high. This increased pressure forces the heart to work harder to pump blood throughout the body. Hypertension affects 50 million Americans, and more than half of men in America over age sixty-five are hypertensive. High blood pressure often has no symptoms, but its consequences are clear. High blood pressure is responsible for a major portion of strokes, heart attacks, kidney failure, and congestive heart disease.

Doctors have traced high blood pressure to high-sodium diets, obesity, alcohol abuse, cigarettes, inactivity, and stress. It can be brought under control with a high-fiber/low-sodium diet, exercise, and medication.

Both upper and lower respiratory tract infections produce fevers, and this increase in body temperature can raise blood pressure. As a result, fever control is especially important if you have hypertension. Although high blood pressure does not increase infection susceptibility per se, hypertension is often accompanied by increased age and related health problems that do depress immunity. The treatment of colds and flu needs to be modified to avoid a rise in blood pressure.

Treatment Issues of Hypertension and Respiratory Infections

ANTI-INFLAMMATORY. Since fever tends to increase blood pressure, these medications are especially important if you have hypertension. Use acetaminophen, ibuprofen, and aspirin regularly as directed on the product package.

ANTIHISTAMINES. All forms of antihistamines can safely be used if you are under age sixty-five with hypertension. Seniors may find that the older sedating antihistamines can cause confusion and loss of balance. For symptom relief, the newer antihistamines that do not cause drowsiness such as Claritin or Allegra can safely relieve sneezing and excess mucus.

VACCINES. Hypertension alone does not put you in the high-risk category for a flu shot, but it probably should. Even if you are young without other health problems, the last thing you want is a week of high fevers from a full-blown case of the flu. Get the flu shot every year, and over age fifty take an additional two minutes at your yearly physical to check if you are up-to-date with your pneumonia vaccination.

ANTIVIRALS. Antiviral drugs can safely be used, but they are not as important as when asthma or COPD are present.

COUGH CONTROL. Be careful to avoid cough products that contain decongestants, which can raise blood pressure. Start with sugar-based lozenges, then move up to syrups that contain dextromethorphan for coughs with phlegm, or guaifenesin for dry coughs. Read the labels carefully to avoid ingredients you don't need.

SUPPLEMENTS. Vitamin C and zinc can be used safely and effectively when high blood pressure is present.

ANTIBIOTICS. Hypertension may lower the threshold for the need for antibiotics to treat bacterial infections that can complicate colds and flu.

NUTRITION. Be careful to use low-sodium chicken soup. Standard canned soups can have over one thousand milligrams of sodium per cup, almost half the total daily recommended intake for hypertension control. If you make your own, avoid adding salt entirely.

HYDROTHERAPY. When you gargle with a saline solution, take care that you rinse thoroughly with cool water and spit out all the rinse water. Rather than relying on a hot shower to dissolve dry, old mucus in the airways, use a tabletop sauna. Fill a bowl with very hot water, put in a few drops of eucalyptus oil, and place on a steady table. Sit down, drape a towel over your head, and breathe in deeply for five minutes.

SENIORS

As the decades go by, the body undergoes changes that increase vulnerability to respiratory infections. The immune response declines, and the body finds it harder to fight off infections. The upper airways are drier, increasing chances that viruses and bacteria can take hold. Gum disease increases chances for bacterial superinfection of a simple viral cold, while nasal polyps produce greater obstruction. The residual damage of past infections and environmental exposures such as cigarette smoke increases the opportunity for simple colds to develop into bronchitis and pneumonia. Social changes also contribute to an increase of infections. Grandparenting is life's reward for being a parent, but grandchildren expose seniors to a steady stream of new viruses.

Respiratory infections can take longer to resolve in seniors. While the usual cold should last five to seven days, in people over age sixty-five, it can take weeks to feel well again. A single severe infection can cause a permanent decline in lung function, so it is important to stay on top of routine infections.

Seniors are more prone to develop sinusitis, especially those caused by a fungus. Each year twenty thousand Americans die from pneumonia, and 90 percent of these deaths are in older people. The increased susceptibility to catching an infection as well as developing complications spur the need to make key changes in the way colds and flu are handled.

Treatment Issues of Seniors and Respiratory Infections

ANTI-INFLAMMATORY. Acetaminophen, ibuprofen, or aspirin can be used safely and effectively to relieve fever and body aches in seniors. Be careful not to exceed recommended dosage since seniors tend to metabolize drugs more slowly. A slower metabolism means that it takes longer for all medications to clear from the blood. To avoid side effects, use the lowest recommended dosage.

ANTIHISTAMINES. Traditional sedating antihistamines are among the most effective for cold relief, but they are not recommended for seniors. They have been shown to cause confusion, disorientation, and dizziness that has led to falls. To relieve sneezing and a runny nose or a respiratory infection, use a second-generation antihistamine such as Claritin or Allegra.

DECONGESTANTS. Incidence of high blood pressure rises as we grow older, and the two major forms of decongestants (phenylephrines and pseudoephedrines) are known to raise blood pressure. Not all seniors have hypertension, and if you don't have hypertension, decongestants should not cause problems. If your blood pressure numbers tend to be higher than normal, use decongestant nasal sprays that contain the anticholinergic ipratropium bromide. These products can shrink blood vessels in the nose without the risk of increasing blood pressure in the rest of the body.

In men over age sixty-five, all forms of decongestants may increase symptoms of prostate disease.

VACCINES. If you are over sixty-five, you are at the top of every list to receive a yearly flu shot. Unfortunately, this immunization is only about 40 percent effective in seniors. In other words, only four out of ten people over sixty-five will get complete flu protection. To improve your odds, studies have now shown that it is more effective to immunize people around you. This includes your friends, coworkers, and family members. It is especially important for your children (and particularly your grandchildren) to be vaccinated against the flu since they turn out to be the leading factors in the rapid spread of the virus.

Most deaths from pneumonia occur in seniors, so pneumonia immunization is equally important and indicated for everyone over age sixty-five.

ANTIVIRALS. If influenza does develop, seniors often do well with antivirals such as Tamiflu. If you have additional risk factors such as lung or heart disease, ask your physician if he recommends having a five-day course of the drug ready at home to be used if flu symptoms appear.

COUGH CONTROL. If you aren't diabetic, start with sugar-based lozenges to coat and soothe an irritated throat. If additional help is needed, use a simple cough medicine without additional antihistamines or decongestants. Codeine-based cough syrups should be reserved for severe coughs of pneumonia or acute exacerbations of COPD, as codeine can cause seniors to become dizzy and lose balance. You don't want to trade a cough for a broken hip.

SUPPLEMENTS. Seniors can use vitamin C and zinc safely and effectively. Do not use supplements of vitamin E or beta-carotene, which may actually increase risk of lung cancers and heart disease.

NUTRITION. Seniors can generally follow the same nutritional advice for adults, but keep age-related health problems in mind. Watch the sodium level of chicken soup if your blood pressure tends to be high. If diabetes is a problem, avoid honey in your hot tea. Seniors tend to be more sensitive to caffeine. Although tea has less than one-third the caffeine found in coffee, over age sixty-five even this level may cause insomnia. To avoid problems, drink decaffeinated tea after 1 p.m. If you feel jittery or have trouble falling asleep, switch to decaffeinated tea at all times.

HYDROTHERAPY. Because of the restrictions on antihistamines and decongestants, water in different forms is especially important for seniors. Relieve nasal congestion with a saline rinse, and wash away viral-laden mucus in the throat with a saline throat gargle. Drink three to four cups of hot tea and lemon as well as several glasses of cold water throughout the day. To avoid slipping or falling, use a rubber mat for hot baths or showers in the tub, and don't take a bath or shower when you are alone at home.

CHAPTER 12

COMMON QUESTIONS
AND ANSWERS

CAUSES OF RESPIRATORY INFECTIONS

1. How does histamine cause problems in colds and other respiratory infections?

Histamine is a natural body chemical that causes blood vessels to dilate and increases production of mucus in the airways. It is well-known that histamine is produced in allergies, but viruses can also provoke their release. These events lead to feelings of congestion and the development of a cough.

2. If birds harbor avian flu virus, can I catch the virus from my parrot?

A number of birds, including chickens, ducks, and geese, have been shown to harbor the avian flu virus. In theory, parrots could be a source of the virus, but it has not been seen in this species of bird. If your pet parrot has lived with you for several years, without contact with other wild birds who may be infected with the virus, it is highly unlikely that Polly could infect you with the avian flu.

3. Are cold sores caused by colds?

Cold sores are caused by the herpes simplex virus, not by one of the over two hundred viruses that lead to colds. People infected with herpes simplex tend to have flare-ups when their immunity is lowered such as during illness or stress. Not infrequently, the herpes infection will cause a mouth sore during or after a bad cold or flu—hence the association and name.

4. Can you get reinfected with a cold? I seem to get better, then my son catches the cold. Next thing I know I've got a cough and fever again.

There are two likely scenarios. The first is that your cold could be developing into sinusitis or bronchitis. These symptoms develop just at the time the original cold symptoms should be fading. Alternatively, your son may have caught a new cold from another source, and one for which you have no immunity. Children catch six to eight colds a year, and they last from ten to fourteen days. It can be hard to know when one cold ends and another begins.

PREVENTING RESPIRATORY INFECTIONS

5. Last year I got the flu shot but I still got the flu. How is that possible?

In general the flu shot is 70–80 percent effective; that is, it provides complete protection 70–80 percent of the time. As we get older, our response to the flu shot declines. Over age seventy, the flu shot may be only 40 percent effective. Sometimes people do not get the flu shot early enough in the year to develop immunity before they are exposed to the virus. In other situations, the flu may have come from a virus not included in the vaccine.

6. Should I stay home from work with a cold?

For your own sake you should stay home if you have a fever. At the start of the cold, if you are sneezing and congested or coughing often, you should stay home to prevent spreading the illness to your coworkers. After two to three days you are shedding less virus and are less likely to infect others.

7. My two-year-old seems to get six colds a year. Is that normal?

Children catch six to eight colds a year, so you're actually doing well.

8. When does a cold become contagious?

In children, colds are contagious one to two days before symptoms begin. In adults, colds are spread once symptoms of sneezing and coughing develop. However in the flu, both children and adults can spread the virus as much as two days before symptoms develop.

9. Should I wear a mask in cold and flu season?

When there is an outbreak of severe infectious disease for which we do not have a vaccine or cure (e.g., SARS), masks are a public health tool to control the spread of the disease. In a routine cold and flu season, wearing a mask is a bit excessive. However, if you have asthma or COPD, the cold air can cause coughing and shortness of breath. I usually recommend wrapping a scarf around the mouth and nose area to warm cold, dry air.

10. How often should I wash my hands to reduce the risk of catching a cold?

Wash your hands if you're exposed to someone with a respiratory infection after using the bathroom, before meals, and before going to bed. The absolute number of washings depends on how many times you perform these activities each day.

11. Are the instant hand sanitizers helpful in reducing colds?

The alcohol-based hand cleansers are practical and easy to use. They have been shown to reduce virus and bacterial levels on the hands. I recommend them after using public telephones and public transportation such as buses and trains. If a coworker clearly has a respiratory infection, using an instant hand wash can reduce your risk of coming down with his or her cold or flu.

12. Are antiseptic sprays helpful in the home and office?

Disinfectant sprays that clean the surface of bathrooms, telephones, and kitchens have been shown to kill both viruses and bacteria. They cannot be used in the air, but cleaning of commonly used surfaces lowers the risk of catching common infections.

13. When am I no longer contagious with a respiratory infection?

An adult can spread a cold for up to six days. You are actually infectious with a flu up to two days before symptoms develop.

DIAGNOSIS OF RESPIRATORY INFECTIONS

14. How can I tell if I have a strep throat?

The symptoms of strep throat are usually more intense than those caused by a virus. Strep throat is usually accompanied by fever and body aches, but sneezing and coughing are absent. To confirm diagnosis, you need a throat culture and RAT test.

15. How can I tell if it's a cold or an allergy?

A cold comes on slowly over six to eight hours. It often begins with a tickle in the throat. Sneezing starts and you feel chilled, congested, and achy. Allergies start suddenly with sneezing and congestion. Body aches, fever, and headaches are usually absent. Allergies often end within a few hours, while colds last five to seven days in adults.

16. When do I need a chest X-ray with a cold or cough?

Normally the three key signs that an X-ray is required are chest pain, shortness of breath, and severe cough accompanied by cloudy green/yellow or rusty mucus. If you have underlying pulmonary or cardiac problems, such as asthma or congestive heart failure, then even without these three symptoms, an X-ray is needed when a respiratory infection lingers beyond five days.

17. Does green phlegm mean I have bronchitis?

Green phlegm is often a sign that a bacterial infection has developed in the airways. It is certainly a signal to call your doctor, but without fever, chest pain, or shortness of breath, it is probably not a danger sign. Green phlegm can also be seen in asthma without any infection.

18. I've read that colds last five to seven days, but I get mini-colds that last less than a day. Is this unusual?

Colds that last for such a short period are probably short-term allergic reactions. True colds caused by viral invasion need time to reproduce and develop fever, cough, and body aches. Antihistamines such as Claritin or Benadryl effectively manage allergic episodes.

TREATMENT ISSUES AND OPTIONS

19. Can vitamin C prevent a cold?

In a word, no. Recent well-designed clinical trials have not shown that vitamin C can prevent colds. However, the same studies indicate that vitamin C may reduce the duration of the symptoms and discomfort.

20. I ran out of pediatric cold medicine. Can I just use less of an adult spray for my two-year-old?

No. This is a dangerous approach. Medication dosages for children are based on their body weight. In addition, adult medications often contain ingredients such as aspirin and alcohol that should not be used in children's medications.

21. How often should I take my temperature?

Always take your temperature before calling a physician, since this is the first question he or she will ask. When you are sick, take your temperature in the morning and evening if you feel feverish to judge how well you are responding to medication or other treatments.

22. If fever is a natural defense against infection, why should I try to lower it?

While fever is a natural part of our defense mechanism, it is not that effective in controlling infections. In fact, fever is dehydrating, raises blood pressure, and puts a strain on the heart and kidneys. You will feel better and recover more quickly if fever is brought under control.

23. Can I use saline rinse for my sore throat if I have high blood pressure?

Saline gargle will not raise blood pressure. You should not absorb harmful levels of sodium while gargling. Be careful to rinse your mouth with cool water after spitting out salty water.

24. Can a mentholated chest rub help me breathe better?

Mentholated rubs give off fumes that stimulate the production of fresh, thin mucus. This fluid helps dissolve old, dry, hardened mucus in your airways, making it easier for you to cough it up or blow it from your nose.

25. Are combination medications more effective than single ingredients?

Combination products offer three distinct advantages. If you take them as directed, you cannot overdose when treating symptoms. In addition, combination products usually are less costly than single ingredients purchased individually. A single product *is also convenient to put in your pocket or purse. On the down-side, combination products may contain ingredients that you don't need or should not use. For example, if you have diabetes, you might need to avoid decongestants, which tend to raise blood sugar levels.*

26. Can I use a decongestant if I have hypertension?

Decongestants improve breathing by narrowing swollen blood vessels in the nose. Unfortunately, decongestants can narrow blood vessels in other parts of the body. Decreasing the diameter of blood vessels makes the heart work harder to pump blood through-out the body. This increased effort can be dangerous.

If your hypertension is well controlled with diet, exercise, and medication, ask your physician if it is safe for you to use deconges-tants.

27. My daughter has had three cases of tonsillitis this year. Should her tonsils be removed?

It's possible. Tonsils used to be routinely removed in small children who had frequent respiratory infections. Doctors believed that by removing the tonsils, new episodes of tonsillitis could be avoided. Currently tonsillectomies are reserved for situations where the tonsils are so enlarged that they cause difficulties in swallowing or breathing.

28. Can I take antibiotics when I'm pregnant?

Physicians would like pregnant women to avoid all medica-tions as much as possible. If a pregnant woman develops a bacterial infection such as severe bronchitis or strep throat, doctors will pre-scribe antibiotics that are known to be safe in pregnancy, including erythromycin or penicillin. Two that should be avoided are tetracy-cline, which causes tooth deformities in the baby, and the quinolones, which cause joint problems in children.

29. My nose always gets so red and raw with a cold or sinus infection. How can I treat it?

The constant wetness and rubbing a nose endures during a cold can leave the tip red and sore. Use a bit of plain Vaseline on the outside of the nostrils to provide a soothing protective coating.

30. Why do menthol or eucalyptus soothe my sore throat? Do they stop viral replication?

Menthol does not have any effect on viral reproduction. In-stead, it acts by temporarily numbing the throat tissue so that pain is lessened.

31. I know that corticosteroids reduce inflammation. Can they help the inflammation of a flu?

Corticosteroids such as prednisone are powerful anti-inflammatory agents, but they do not reduce symptoms of colds and flus. However, they are prescribed for some types of severe life-threatening infections such as SARS and acute exacerbations of COPD.

32. Why do antihistamines make me so sleepy?

Antihistamines cross the blood-brain barrier and depress the action of the center in the brain that causes alertness.

ALTERNATIVE HEALTH TREATMENTS AND RESPIRATORY INFECTIONS

33. My Chinese grandmother uses acupuncture for colds. How does it work?

Acupuncture is a traditional form of Chinese medicine that relies on "adjusting the balance of energies between organs." Acupuncture practitioners have mapped out links and points in the body and stimulate these areas with fine needles to control disease and relieve symptoms. Research has shown that acupuncture needles at a point in the lower back provide some relief to blocked bronchi. Some people respond better than others to acupuncture. In China today, acupuncture needles are used in conjunction with Western medicine.

34. Is garlic good for colds?

Garlic has mild antibacterial activity, but it is not strong enough to help you fight off infections such as strep throat or bacterial bronchitis. Garlic is delicious in food, but you need more targeted treatments for these problems.

35. My aunt used to wrap a sore throat with a warm scarf—it seemed to help. How does that work?

The air that passes through the throat is cool and dry, which is irritating to the airways. The scarf warms the throat, which in turn warms the air inside.

36. Can a mustard plaster break up chest congestion?

The fumes from the mustard plaster stimulate increased mucus production in the airways. This fresh, thin mucus dilutes the dried, hardened mucus that has accumulated in the airways. As a result, it is easier to blow your nose and cough up the mucus.

37. Can honey help a cough or sore throat?

Honey is a "demulcent"—it creates a coating on the throat that soothes irritation. Adding a teaspoon of honey to a cup of hot tea makes a soothing beverage even better.

NUTRITION AND RESPIRATORY INFECTIONS

38. Should you feed a cold and starve a fever?

You need both nutrients and fluids to combat any illness. A fever actually dehydrates the body and increases the need for liquids. If the flu has upset the gastrointestinal tract, hot tea, chicken soup, and ice cream provide both fluids and calories during the acute phase.

39. Can I drink alcohol with a cold or flu?

Alcohol is a vasodilator, meaning that it expands blood vessels. This means it can actually add to feelings of congestion. You should avoid beer, wine, and spirits for the duration of the illness. However, adding a teaspoon of cognac or brandy to a cup of hot tea will help you relax and get a good night's sleep.

40. Does milk increase mucus production?

If you have a milk allergy, dairy products may increase congestion. But if you can consume dairy products without problems, they will not increase mucus production during a respiratory illness.

41. Why do I lose my sense of smell and taste when I have a cold?

During a cold, the mucus coating on the airways combined with inflammation of the mouth and nasal passages block and deaden the nerves involved with taste and smell.

42. I'm a vegetarian. Is vegetable soup as effective as chicken soup?

Vegetable soup has some anti-inflammatory properties, but not nearly as much as soup made with chicken.

43. Is green tea better against colds and flu than standard tea?

Green tea is higher in antioxidants than black tea, but in the case of respiratory infections, black tea has additional benefits. It contains theobromine, which helps keep airways open. This relieves congestion and tightness in the chest, helping you to breathe easier.

44. I have diabetes. I shouldn't drink OJ. Is there any other way to get vitamin C?

You can get vitamin C naturally in grapefruit, red peppers, and strawberries. To combat a cold, take 250–500 milligrams of extra vitamin C per day. Keep in mind that excessive vitamin C supplements can cause diarrhea and acid reflux.

45. Is it okay to smoke while sick with a cold or flu?

That's a really loaded question. It's never healthy to smoke, and it's particularly harmful during a respiratory infection. Cigarette smoke paralyzes the cilia, tiny hairlike structures in the airways that sweep out mucus and bacteria. This increases congestion as well as the severity and length of the illness. Smokers have more symptoms and their colds last longer.

Actually a bad cold or flu is an excellent time to quit smoking. Use a nicotine patch to deal with the cravings. By the time the cough and fever have gone, you can be on your way to living as an ex-smoker.

LIFESTYLE RESPIRATORY ISSUES

46. Is it okay to wash my hair when I have a cold?

A warm shower actually helps dissolve mucus in both the upper and lower airways, but don't go outside with wet hair. Although clinical studies have shown that soaking and chilling healthy volunteers did not cause colds, the additional chill can cause a physically stressful situation that may depress the immune response.

47. Do humidifiers prevent colds?

Humidifiers don't actually prevent colds, but once a respiratory infection has developed, humidifiers may help. Cold, dry air can increase both discomfort and the risk of developing sinusitis. By adding moisture to the air, humidifiers reduce dryness and decrease the chances of complications, especially in children.

48. Should I fly with a cold?

It is not the best idea to fly with a respiratory infection. The pressurized cabin can force mucus into the sinus cavities and fluid into the eustachian tubes, thereby spreading the infection. In addition, the extremely dry air in the cabin will increase irritation of your airways. If you must travel, use a decongestant be-

fore taking off and drink plenty of fluids, including hot tea, dur-
ing the flight.

49. Should I exercise with a cold?

I suggest that you do a "neck check." If your symptoms are
above your neck (e.g., sneezing, congestion, or sore throat), then it's
okay to work out. But if you have symptoms below the neck, in-
cluding cough, body aches, and chills, then take a break from the
gym.

50. Does stress cause me to catch colds?

Repeated studies have shown that stress depresses immunity
and may increase your risk of developing infections. Unfortunately,
it's easy to tell you to relax, and much harder to control the work
and family relationships that are stressful. In peak season for colds
and flu, try to break the stress buildup by taking time for yourself.
Once a day do something that is all about you. Read a magazine
or a book, watch a favorite TV show, or meet friends to help you
regroup.

51. When should I call the doctor?

With most respiratory infections you probably feel sicker than
you are. Nasal congestion makes it hard to breathe, while inflam-
matory compounds raise your fever and produce aches and fatigue.
But despite your discomfort, you're probably not that ill. When
you call your physician with these complaints, you are not likely to
get much sympathy. However, three clear signals to call your doctor
are:

- Temperature 102° F or higher
- Chest pain
- Shortness of breath

These are symptoms that indicate a significant infection has developed in your respiratory system and prompt medical attention is needed.

In addition to dramatic symptoms, it is important to call your physician if cold and flu symptoms continue past seven days in an adult. This could be a sign that sinusitis or bronchitis has developed, and targeted medication may be needed.

52. Why don't doctors get colds?

Doctor's do get colds and flu, but probably less frequently than would be expected from their repeated exposures, but we don't really know why. Exposure to a great number of viruses may ultimately lead to greater protection, as may greater adherence to hygiene precautions. A form of self-selection known as the "healthy worker effect" may also play a role. This suggests that people who stay in a given type of job for long periods are better suited physiologically and immunologically to not get ill in that environment. This concept has been used to explain why some older workers in dusty industries seem to have fewer respiratory problems than predicted from the responses of young workers coming into the industry.

SMOKING AND RESPIRATORY INFECTIONS

53. Can I smoke marijuana with a cold?

An urban legend is that marijuana smoke is less harmful than traditional tobacco smoke. Actually, marijuana is more irritating to the airways than cigarettes. One study indicated that a single marijuana joint delivers as much as four times the amount of tar as a filtered cigarette.

54. My husband is a heavy smoker who is getting over pneumonia. Can he use the nicotine patch to help him quit smoking?

Nicotine patches will help keep your husband comfortable. A severe illness is often the critical moment when an individual has the right motivation and circumstances to help him or her quit smoking.

55. Why do cigarettes taste so much better when I have a cold?

You lose your sense of smell and taste during an upper respiratory infection, so you don't sense just how raw and nasty the tobacco tastes.

56. Do smokers get more colds?

Smokers don't necessarily get more colds, but their infections last longer and are much more likely to develop into sinusitis, bronchitis, and even pneumonia.

57. Since menthol is found in cold remedies, should I switch to menthol cigarettes when I become congested?

Menthol is an effective decongestant, but in cigarettes it's meant to counteract the irritation and odor of tobacco. It's a bad use of an effective ingredient.

INDEX

acetaminophen, 32–34, 71, 72, 80, 91,
    124
  for bronchitis, 100, 104
  for children, 178, 180, 188, 194
  individual needs and, 197, 199, 203,
    205, 209, 211, 213
  for influenza, 156, 172, 173, 188
  for pleurisy, 98–99
  for pneumonia, 143, 147
acetylcholine, 30, 36
acetylcysteine, 143
aches, body, 31, 62, 197, 220, 229
  cold and, 7, 31, 64
  influenza and, 156, 158, 168, 172, 187
acupuncture, 225
addiction, 29
adenoids, 13, 14, 15
adenovirus, 61, 63, 145, 184, 195
Advair, 111
advanced age, 9, 33, 46, 62
  individual needs and, 197, 212–15
  influenza and, 157, 162, 170, 214–15,
    217
  pneumonia and, 67, 142–43, 168, 171,
    213
  vaccination and, 40, 45, 46, 142–43,
    162, 214
Advil, 33, 71
Advisory Committee on Immunization
    Practices (ACIP), 205
Afrin spray, 29
air conditioning, 22, 23, 110, 130

airways:
  basic jobs of, 16
  bronchitis and, 94, 95, 95, 96, 103
  coughs and, 34–36
  lower, 6, 12, 15, 16–17, 36, 37, 66, 84,
    102
  upper, 6, 11–17, 13, 20, 36, 37, 84, 86,
    147
albuterol, 36, 100, 112
alcohol, alcohol abuse, 21, 32, 33, 130,
    206, 221, 226
  pneumonia and, 140, 141
Allegra, 28, 91, 211, 214
allergies, 7, 12, 30, 75, 97, 114, 226
  to antibiotics, 38, 39, 80, 124, 183
  in children, 177, 179–80, 181, 183,
    191, 199
  colds vs., 61, 66, 220, 221
  histamine and, 17, 28, 216
  sinusitis and, 84, 85, 89, 90, 91, 93
  to sulfa drugs, 80
  treatment of, 28, 49, 89, 93, 221
  triggering of, 84, 89
alpha agonists, 29
alveoli, 16–17
  pneumonia and, 128, 131, 133, 134,
    137, 138, 145
amantadine, 46–47
American Academy of Pediatrics,
    121–22
American College of Physicians, 99, 119
American Heart Association, 121–22

American Medical Association, 36
American Thoracic Society (ATS), 36, 108, 138–39
amoxicillin, 38, 80, 88, 181, 183, 186, 194
amphotericin, 87–88
analgesics, 35
    see also aspirin; Tylenol
Anaprox, 199
antibiotics, 24, 36–39, 72
    for bronchitis, 34, 39, 99, 100, 102, 104–5, 112, 116
    children and, *see* children, antibiotics and
    combining of, 21, 22, 24
    coughs and, 34
    "designer," 20, 37–38
    individual needs and, 200, 204, 207, 210, 212
    for influenza, 156, 172, 173, 189
    length of therapy with, 22
    for mycoplasma, 26, 150, 151
    for pneumonia, 26, 34, 128, 143, 146, 147, 150, 151, 184, 186, 187
    pregnancy and, 223–24
    resistance to, 11, 18, 20, 21–22, 37, 83, 89, 99, 102, 118, 187
    for sinusitis, 38, 39, 79, 80, 88–89, 92
    for sinusitis complications, 82, 83
    for sore throats, 117
    for strep throat, 8, 39, 117, 118, 123, 124
    types of, 37–39
    see also erythromycin; penicillin
antibodies, 25, 40, 42–43, 126, 149, 159, 175–76, 191
anticholinergics, 30, 36
anticoagulants, 83
antigenic drift, 40, 159
antigenic shift, 40, 159
antihistamines, 100, 147, 173, 221, 224
    for children, 178, 180–81, 194
    colds and, 27–28, 34, 35, 55, 71, 72, 178
    individual needs and, 199, 203, 206, 209, 211, 213–14, 215
    sinusitis and, 80, 89, 91
anti-inflammatory treatment, 124
    for bronchitis, 100, 104, 112, 116, 168
    for colds and flu, 31–34, 47–48, 55, 72, 227
    individual needs and, 199, 203, 205, 209, 211, 213
    for influenza, 156, 172, 173, 188, 224

for pneumonia, 143, 147
    for sinusitis, 7, 80, 91, 93
antileukotrienes, 89, 91
antioxidants, 48, 55, 201, 209–10, 227
antiseptic sprays, 219
antiviral medications, 9, 73, 80, 191
    bronchitis and, 99, 101, 105
    individual needs and, 200, 203, 206, 209, 211, 214–15
    for influenza, 156, 157, 172, 173, 188
    for pneumonia, 144, 147, 148
anxiety, 47, 48
appetite, loss of, 145, 176, 179, 192
aromatic chemicals, 30
arteries, plaque formation in, 22
Asian flu (1957), 158, 160–61, 162
aspirin, 7, 31–35, 48, 71, 72, 80, 91, 124
    asthma and, 32, 197, 199, 209
    for bronchitis, 100, 104
    children and, 32, 41, 169, 170, 177–78, 187–88, 221
    individual needs and, 199, 203, 205, 209, 211, 213
    for influenza, 156, 172, 173
    for pneumonia, 143, 147
asthma, 5, 8, 9, 30, 47, 72, 157, 218, 220
    airway muscles and, 17
    aspirin and, 32, 197, 199, 209
    bronchitis and, 96, 102, 168
    bronchitis compared with, 96, 97
    causes of, 26
    in children, 177, 185, 188, 191, 199
    coughs compared with, 35–36
    diet and, 109, 201
    individual needs and, 197–201
    influenza and, 167, 172, 173, 200
    sinusitis and, 84
    triggers for, 17, 22, 32, 67, 69, 198
    vaccines and, 41, 46, 172, 200
Atrovent, 30, 36, 100, 104, 111, 112
Augmentin, 38, 79, 80, 88, 92, 104–5, 143, 173
autism, 44, 188
Avelox, 39
Aventis, 42, 170
avian (bird) flu, 40, 45, 67, 160, 163–65, 216
Awakenings (Sacks), 155

bacteremia, 21, 141
bacteria, 12, 14, 17–24, 34, 36–39, 227
    antibiotic-resistant, 11, 18, 20, 21–22, 37, 83, 89, 99, 102, 118, 187

bronchitis and, *see* bronchitis, acute
   bacterial
cilia and, 6, 14, 76, 106, 140
classification of, 18–23
coexistence and, 17–18
croup and, 195
flu vaccine contaminated with, 41, 42
hydrotherapy and, 49–51
mycoplasma compared with, 26
pneumonia and, *see* pneumonia,
   bacterial
sinusitis and, 20, 21, 22, 67, 75–84,
   88–89, 200
strep throat and, 118–23
viruses compared with, 24, 120
Bactrim, 80
Baxter International, 44–45
Bayer pharmaceutical company, 31
Benadryl, 28, 221
benzocaine, 35, 72, 124, 173
beta agonists, 36, 100
beta-carotene, 109–10, 210, 215
Beta-Carotene and Retinol Efficiency
   Study (CARET), 109–10
beta lactams, 37–38, 39
   see also penicillin
Biaxin, 39, 124, 151, 173
birth defects, 177, 205–7
blindness, 82, 201
blood clots, blood clotting, 56, 83, 98,
   136, 137
blood culture, 135
blood disease, chronic, 41
blood pressure:
   high, *see* hypertension
   increase in, 29, 33, 56, 126, 178, 199,
      206, 209, 210–12, 214, 222
blood sugar, 83, 201–3, 223
blood tests, 103, 149
blood vessels, 71, 96, 132, 201, 226
   shrinking of, 29, 30
bradykinins, 63–64, 114
brain, 34, 155, 167, 224
brain abscess, 83, 142
breastbone, 16
breath, shortness of, 98, 126, 137, 151,
   167, 220, 229–30
   bronchitis and, 106, 107, 113, 114,
      115, 220
   individual needs and, 200, 202, 208–9
   in pneumonia, 130, 131–32, 145, 168,
      169
bronchi, 6, *15*, 16, 64, 96, 128, 166

bronchial tree, *15*, 16
bronchiolitis, 67, 190–91
bronchitis, 2, 7–8, 16, 34, 66, 94–117,
   202, 213, 217, 231
   acute, 8, 9, 65
   in children, 177, 181–82
   influenza and, 156, 168, 172, 173
bronchitis, acute bacterial, 39, 94, 102–5,
   200
   causes of, 21, 22, 102–3
bronchitis, acute viral, 94–102
   causes of, 61, 67, 95–96
   diagnosis of, 97–99
   impact of infection in, 96
   prevention of, 99
   symptoms of, 95, 138
   transmission of, 96
   treatment for, 99–102
bronchitis, chronic, 8, 69, 94
   acute exacerbation of, 94–95, 112–16
   causes of, 106–7
   diagnosis of, 107–8
   prevention of, 108–10
   transmission of, 107
   treatment of, 110–13
bronchodilators, 2, 48, 144, 191, 200
   anticholinergic, 30, 36
   beta-agonist, 36, 100
   bronchitis and, 2, 100, 104, 105,
      110–11, 112, 116

caffeine, 48, 215
cancer, 109, 215
carbon dioxide, 16, 17, 128, 133
carriage, 183
carrier state, 8
cavernous sinus, 83
Ceclor, 38
Ceftin, 38, 143, 194
Celsus, 3
Centers for Disease Control and
   Prevention (CDC), 36, 67, 74, 99,
   107, 115, 121, 185, 205
   influenza and, 40, 161–62
central nervous system, 24, 142, 206
cephalosporins, 38, 181, 187
chemotherapy, 46, 142, 172
chest, 16, 34, 222
   pain in, *see* pain, chest
chest X-rays, 65, 97–98, 190, 220
   for bronchitis, 103, 107, 115
   for pneumonia, 127, 128, *132*, *133*, 134,
      136–38, 140, 145, *146*, 149, 184

chicken pox, 169, 178
chicken soup, 47–48, 71–72, 73, 81, 92, 125, 151, 226, 227
  individual needs and, 207, 212, 215
Childhood Immunization Act (1992), 43
children, 6, 9, 20, 21, 175–96
  allergies in, 177, 179–80, 181, 183, 191, 199
  antibiotics and, 37, 126, 179, 181, 183, 184, 186, 187, 189, 194
  aspirin and, 32, 41, 169, 170, 177–78, 187–88, 221
  asthma in, 177, 185, 188, 191, 199
  autism in, 44, 188
  bronchiolitis in, 67, 190–91
  bronchitis in, 177, 181–82
  colds in, 9, 25, 57–61, 68, 175–79, 182, 192, 217, 218, 221
  croup in, 61, 67, 190, 194–96
  earaches in, 15, 176–77, 185, 187, 189, 190, 192–94
  humidifiers for, 50, 179, 228
  influenza in, 9, 57–58, 158, 160, 161, 163, 164, 169, 170, 171, 182, 187–89, 192, 218
  pneumonia in, 67, 130, 145, 177, 184–87
  Reye's syndrome in, 32, 169, 177–78, 188
  rheumatic fever in, 126, 183
  RSV infection in, 25–26, 61, 145, 184, 190, 191
  sinusitis in, 7, 179–81
  strep throat in, 117, 122, 123, 126, 182–84
  tonsils of, 14, 182, 183–84, 223
  vaccines for, see vaccines, for children
chills, 98, 119, 129, 145, 149, 169, 220, 229
China, 154, 158–59, 163, 225
  SARS in, 61, 62
Chiron, 45, 170
chlamydia, 8, 136
Chlamydia pneumoniae, 22
chlorpheniramine (Chlor-Trimeton), 28
cilia, 6, 12–13, 14, 17, 145
  in sinuses, 75, 76
  smoking and, 14, 85, 106, 140, 227
Claritin, 28, 91, 211, 214, 221
clavulanic acid, 38, 88
clemastine (Tavist), 28
Cleveland Clinic, 52

Clinical Laboratories Improvement Act (1988), 121
codeine, 34, 100, 104, 112, 143, 147, 173, 178
  individual needs and, 200, 203–4, 206, 215
coffee, 48, 215
cold air, 35–36, 84, 196, 218, 228
colds, 59–73, 117, 216–21, 224–31
  allergies vs., 61, 66, 220, 221
  causes of, 3, 7, 60–63, 76, 145, 216, 217, 229
  chest vs. head, 98
  in children, 9, 25, 57–61, 68, 175–79, 182, 192, 217, 218, 221
  cilia and, 6, 13, 14
  complications of, 65–68, 94, 95, 96, 98, 176–77
  diagnosis of, 65, 220
  economic impact of, 2, 59–60
  geography of, 69
  history of, 2–4
  immunity to, 68
  impact of infection in, 63–64
  imprecise use of term, 2
  incidence of, 2, 59
  inflammation of, 7, 15, 27, 28, 29, 31–34, 47–48, 63–64, 72
  influenza vs., 157–58
  "old-time" home remedies for, 71
  old wives tales about, 64, 65, 68
  prevention of, 7, 69–70, 96, 205, 218–19, 221, 228
  symptoms of, 1, 2–3, 7, 9, 11, 28, 60, 63–66, 157, 176
  time of the month for, 70
  transmission of, 7, 63, 70, 176, 218, 219
  treatment for, 2, 3, 6–7, 9, 11, 27–39, 47–58, 71–73, 93, 177–79, 199, 200, 203, 211–12, 221, 225, 226
  vocabulary of, 60
  see also influenza
cold sores, 217
combination drugs, 32–33, 222–23
Common Cold Unit, 4
congestion, 13, 18, 64, 66, 118, 119–20, 130, 216, 218, 220, 229
  bronchitis and, 94, 95, 96
  in children, 182, 185, 187, 192
  influenza and, 156, 172, 173
  rebound, 29, 30, 173
  sinusitis and, 85, 89

treatment for, 28, 48–49, 50, 71–72, 73, 101, 173, 215, 225–26, *see also* decongestants
congestive heart failure, 33, 136–37, 210, 220
Congress, U.S., 43–44
Cook, James, 54
Coopersmith, Peggy Sue, 153
COPD (chronic obstructive pulmonary disease), 47, 72, 106, 173, 218, 224
   individual needs and, 197, 208–10
   vaccines and, 41, 46
corn syrup, 35
coronaviruses, 25, 61, 62, 63
corticosteroids, 191, 196, 200, 224
cough drops, 35, 72, 182, 203
coughs, 4–8, 11, 14, 119–20, 216, 220, 229
   bronchitis and, 94, 95, 97, 98, 100, 104, 105, 106, 112, 113, 115, 117, 168, 182
   in children, 182, 185, 186, 187, 194
   colds and, 2, 6, 28, 34–36, 60, 62–66, 68, 69, 72, 218
   individual needs and, 200, 203–4, 206, 211–12, 215
   influenza and, 4, 28, 153, 156, 157, 158, 167, 172, 173, 187
   pleurisy and, 98
   pneumonia and, 117, 129–31, 143, 145, 147, 148, 149, 168, 185, 186, 187
   treatment for, 28, 34–36, 48, 91, 100, 104, 105, 143, 147, 172, 173, 182, 200, 203–4, 206, 211–12, 215, 226
cough sprays, 35
cough suppressants (antitussives), 34, 72, 99, 104, 112, 173, 200
Coxsackie virus, 61, 63, 145
croup, 61, 67, 190, 194–96
CT scans, 7, 77, 82, 83, 86, 180
cystic fibrosis, 185, 188, 191
cytokines, 7, 18, 64, 71, 166, 172
Czech Republic, vaccine production in, 44–45

dairy products, 226
Davis, Katherine, 1–2
Davis, Nate, 1
day care centers, 123, 180, 192
decongestants, 9, 29–30, 48, 147, 223, 229
   for bronchitis, 100
   for children, 178, 181, 194
   for colds, 34, 35, 55, 71, 72, 178

individual needs and, 199, 203, 206, 209, 214, 215
   for influenza, 173
   sinusitis and, 79, 80, 89, 91
dehydration, 33, 222, 226
demulcents, 35, 226
dextromethorphan, 34, 35, 72, 100, 104, 173, 178, 200, 206
diabetes, 5, 67, 102, 109, 172, 227
   individual needs and, 197, 201–4, 215
   vaccines and, 41, 46, 142, 169, 172, 203
diarrhea, 38, 55, 56, 176, 227
diet, 109, 110, 113, 223, 226–27
   see also nutritional therapy
diphenhydramine, 28
DNase, 120
doctors:
   colds of, 230
   when to call, 229–30
doorknobs, 26, 63
drowsiness, 28, 211, 224
Duff, Emily, 117
Duff, Gordon, 117, 122

ear, nose, and throat (ENT) specialists, 85–86, 89, 90
earaches, 15, 176–77, 185, 187, 190, 192–94
   causes of, 20, 21, 192
   flu shots and, 189, 193
eardrum, *13*, 15
ears, 6, 147
   middle, 15, 37, 192, 193
echinacea, 51–52, 200
echovirus, 63
eczema, 97, 180
Egypt, ancient, 2, 54
elderberry, *55*–56
emphysema, 30, 69, 137–38, 168, 208
empyema, 141
encephalitis, 155
endocarditis, chronic, 155
England, 4, 31, 52, 170, 171
environmental irritation, 208
   bronchitis and, 94, 95–96, 106, 110, 114, 168
   see also smoking, smoke, secondhand
Environmental Protection Agency, 110
epinephrine, 196
Epstein-Barr virus, 123
erythromycin, 20, 39, 150, 183, 186, 187, 207, 223

esophagus, stomach acid refluxed into, 97
ethmoid sinus, *13*, 74–75, 76
eucalyptus, 30, 101, 224
Europe:
    supplements in, 51
    vaccine production in, 44–45
eustachian tubes, *13*, 15, 176–77, 193,
    228
exercise, 109, 111, 113, 223, 229
exhaustion, 34, 35
    influenza and, 153, 156, 157, 158, 166,
    172
expectorants, 34–35
eyes, 63, 156
    pain around, 65, 66
    sinusitis complications and, 82, 83

fatigue, 18, 82, 88, 151, 229
fever, 18, 62, 137, 141, 202, 210–11,
    211, 229
    bronchitis and, 100, 102, 103, 104,
    115, 168, 172, 182, 220
    in children, 182, 185–88, 192, 194
    colds and, 3, 7, 31–34, 60, 64, 66, 68,
    69, 71, 218
    influenza and, 153, 156, 158, 166–67,
    172, 173, 187, 188
    pneumonia and, 127, 130, 135, 138,
    143, 145, 149, 168, 169, 185, 186
    sinusitis and, 77, 88
    sinusitis complications and, 82, 83
    strep throat and, 120, 122, 124, 220
    treatment for, 32, 33, 37, 47, 49, 71,
    173, 197, 222, 226
Fexofenadine, 28
Flonase, 90
Flovent, 100, 112
flu, *see* influenza
fluconazole, 87–88
fluids:
    intake of, 47, 101, 179, 226, 229
    retention of, 33
    see also specific fluids
FluMist, 189
flu shots, *see* vaccine, influenza
Fluticasone, 91, 180
Fluvirin, 188
flying, 82, 228–29
fomites, 63
Food and Drug Administration (FDA),
    42, 43, 44
Ford, Gerald, 162
Franklin, Ben, 3

free radicals, 33, 48, 55, 201
Friedman, Jack, 11–12
frontal sinus, *13*, 74–75, 76
Fujian strain, 40, 158, 163
fungal sinusitis, 88

garlic, 225
gastrointestinal problems, 32, 38, 47, 48,
    176, 187
genetic drift, 25, 40, 159
genetic shifts, 159, 160, 167
GERD (gastroesophageal reflux disease),
    97
Germany, 51
glomerulonephritis, 20, 118, 119, 126
Glucophage, 202
glycerin, 35
goldenseal, 56
Gram's stain, 18, 103, 129, 135
Greece, ancient, 2–3, 54, 154
guaifenesin, 35, 206
Guillian-Barre syndrome, 162–63

Haemophilus influenzae (Hib), 21, 76, 130,
    136, 185, 192, 195
    vaccine for, 195, 196
hair, washing of, 228
handrails, 26, 63
hands:
    shaking of, 63, 81
    washing of, 7, 69–70, 79, 96, 99, 123,
    152, 187, 205, 219
hand sanitizers, 219
headache, 14, 82, 119, 145, 158, 182, 220
    migraine, 78
    sinusitis and, 77, 78, 84, 91
    sinusitis complications and, 82, 83
    treatment for, 31, 33–34, 71, 91
"healthy worker effect," 230
heart attacks, 22, 137, 201, 210
heartburn, 48, 97
heart disease, 5, 8, 102, 109, 110, 172,
    214–15
    in children, 177, 191
    chronic, 41, 46
    influenza and, 155, 167
    pneumonia and, 130, 134, 142
    rheumatic, 20, 118, 119, 122, 125–26,
    183
heart failure, congestive, 33, 136–37,
    210, 220
heart rate, increase in, 29, 36, 199
hemagglutinin (H), 160, *161*, 166

hemoglobin, 139
hemolytic anemia, 151
hemolytic staph, 19
HEPA air filters, 96, 110, 111, 113
hepatitis, 32
herpes simplex, 23, 24, 217
Hippocrates, 2–3, 141, 154
histamine, 17, 27–28, 63, 64, 89, 93, 216
HIV, 41, 142, 172
honey, 35, 48, 72, 101, 125, 182, 215, 226
Hong Kong flu (1968), 40, 158, 161, 162
hospitals, hospitalization, 21, 22, 26, 38,
    62, 115, 116, 137, 187, 208
  emergency room of, 195, 196
  intensive care unit of, 139
  pneumonia and, 9, 128, 138–39, 143,
    144, 146–47, 148, 184
humidifiers, 50–51, 92, 101, 105, 125,
    144, 148, 151, 179, 228
humidity, 50–51
humming, 7, 88
hydrotherapy, 49–51, 73, 81, 92
  for bronchitis, 101, 113
  for children, 179, 181, 195
  individual needs and, 201, 207, 212, 215
  for pneumonia, 144, 148
hygrometer, 50
hypertension (high blood pressure), 9,
    33, 109, 222, 223
  individual needs and, 197, 209–12,
    214, 215

ibuprofen, 7, 33, 71, 72, 80, 91, 99, 124
  for bronchitis, 100, 104
  for children, 178, 180, 188, 194
  individual needs and, 199, 203, 205,
    209, 211, 213
  for influenza, 156, 172, 173, 188
  for pneumonia, 143, 147
ice cream, 48, 49, 204, 226
ice packs, 49, 92, 181
immune system, 4, 6, 142, 202
  bacteria and, 18, 120, 126
  of children, 9, 126
immunoassay, 8
impetigo, 119
Infectious Disease Society of America, 122
inflammation, inflammatory compounds,
    29, 31–34, 167, 183, 229
  of bronchi, see bronchitis
  characteristics of, 27
  colds and, 7, 15, 27, 28, 29, 31–34,
    47–48, 63–64, 72

influenza and, 15, 156, 172, 173
  pneumonia and, 130–33, 141, 145
  sinusitis and, 84, 86, 87, 89, 90, 93
  see also cytokines; histamine;
    interleukins
influenza (flu), 2–7, 14, 65, 117, 153–74,
    226–28
  A, 25, 46–47, 158, 159
  B, 25, 46, 47, 157, 158, 159
  C, 25, 157, 158
  causes of, 21, 25, 158–60
  in children, 9, 57–58, 158, 160, 161,
    163, 164, 169, 170, 171, 182,
    187–89, 192, 218
  colds vs., 157–58
  complications of, 94, 95, 96, 155, 156,
    161, 168–69, 172
  deaths from, 2, 5, 45, 67, 154–56,
    159–64, 169, 187
  diagnosis of, 167
  drugs for, 46–47
  early warning system for, 160–64
  genetic drift and, 25, 40
  history of, 4–5
  impact on body of, 166–67
  inflammation of, 15, 156, 172, 173
  old wives tales about, 64, 65, 68
  pandemics of, 3–5, 23, 24, 45, 154–56,
    158–64, 169
  pregnancy and, 205, 206
  prevention of, 9, 96, 146, 147, 169–70,
    188–89, 217–18
  reverse genetics and, 164–65
  symptoms of, 4, 156–58, 165, 166–67,
    187
  transmission of, 165–66, 218,
    219
  treatment for, 6–7, 11, 28, 31–34,
    36–37, 39–58, 172–74, 187–88,
    199, 200, 203, 206, 209, 211–12,
    214–15, 224
  vaccine for, see vaccine, influenza
insomnia, 29, 36, 46, 215
insulin, 201, 202
Intal, 89, 91
interferon, 51
interleukins, 18, 114, 172
intracellular adhesion molecule
    (ICAM–1), 52

jitteriness, 29, 47, 215
juice, 47, 81, 101, 105
  orange, 54–55, 73, 174, 204, 227

kidney disease, 8, 20, 118, 119, 122
  chronic, 41, 46
kidney failure, 22–23, 62, 201, 210
kidney problems, 33, 155, 167, 222
kinins (mediators), 63–64, 71
kissing, 64
klebsiella, 21, 136
Koch, Robert, 3

LAIV (trivalent live, attenuated
    influenza), 40
larynx (voice box), 13, 15
Learner, Harry, 114
Legionella pneumophila (Legionnaire's
    bacillus), 22–23, 130
lemon, 48, 101, 125, 182, 215
leukotrienes, 64, 89, 93
Levaquin, 39, 79, 80, 88, 92, 104–5, 143,
    151
Lewis, David, 161–62
Listerine cough control, 35
liver damage, 32, 155, 167
loratadine, 28
lozenges, 35, 124, 173, 182, 206, 215
  zinc, 53, 73, 200, 204
lung cancer, 109, 215
lung disease, 130, 142, 191, 214–15
  chronic, 21, 41, 46, 109
  see also asthma; COPD
lungs, 6, 14, 15, 16, 24, 37, 62, 84, 98
  abcesses in, 19
  bronchiolitis and, 190
  bronchitis and, 2, 8, 94, 97, 108, 109,
    115
  influenza and, 155
  interstitium of, 133
  lobes of, 15, 16, 137
  pneumonia and, 8, 22, 128, 129, 131,
    137, 168–69, 184
  spirometry and, 97, 108, 115
Lysol, 70

macrolides, 39, 151, 187
marijuana, 230
masks, 218
mast cell inhibitors, 89, 91
maxillary sinus, 13, 74–75, 76, 77
meningitis, 20, 21, 43, 82–83, 142
menstrual cycle, 70
menthol, 30, 224, 231
metformin, 202
microscopes, 18, 20, 23–24, 160
middle ear, 15, 37, 192, 193

military, 43, 60, 122, 123, 155, 161–62
Miller, Thomas, 127, 149
molds, 84, 110, 179
mononucleosis, 123
Motrin, 33
MRI (magnetic resonance imaging), 86,
    87
muccociliary system, 140
mucous membranes, 12–15, 17, 24, 84
  bacteria and, 19, 20
mucus, 12–15, 37, 97, 215, 227
  bronchitis and, 94, 95, 95, 100, 103,
    105, 106, 111, 114, 168, 172, 182
  coughing and, 130–31
  hardening and accumulation of, 13, 14,
    30, 34, 76, 79, 103–4, 222, 226
  histamines and, 17, 28
  pneumonia and, 130, 135, 140, 143,
    144, 145, 148, 169
  sinusitis and, 76, 77, 79, 80, 81, 86, 93,
    181
  stimulation of production of, 30, 48,
    64
  thinning of, 47, 48–49, 71–72, 81, 222,
    225–26
mucus culture, 135
mustard, 30, 225–26
mycoplasma, 8, 26, 129, 149–52, 186–87
myocardium, 125

nasal septum, 12, 13
nasal sprays, 40, 181
  as decongestants, 29–30, 72, 79, 91,
    100
  for sinusitis, 79, 81, 82, 91, 92
  zinc, 53, 81, 82
nasopharynx, 13, 14, 75, 79
National Center for Health Statistics, 74
National Headache Foundation, 78
National Health Survey, 59
National Public Health Institute, Finish,
    109
National Vaccine Injury Compensation
    Program (1986), 43–44
Native Americans, 3, 51, 56
nausea, 38, 56, 156, 159, 182, 187
  zinc and, 53, 54
nebulizers, 50, 88, 181
"neck check," 229
neuraminidase (N), 160, 161
neuraminidase inhibitors, 47
neutrophils, 48, 72
nicotine patches, 228, 231

nonsteroidal anti-inflammatories
    (NSAIDs), 33, 199
nose, 6, 12–14, *13*, 19, 24, 37, 63, 84, 85,
    224
    cilia in, 6, 12–13, 14, 85
    runny, 2, 6
    shrinking of blood vessels in, 29, 30
    stuffy, 60, 157
nursing homes, 41, 46, 129, 169, 171
nutritional therapy, 47–49, 71–72, 73
    for bronchitis, 101, 105, 113
    for children, 179, 181
    individual needs and, 201, 204, 207,
        212, 215
    for influenza, 174
    for pneumonia, 144, 148
    for sinusitis, 81, 92, 181
    for strep throat, 125

orbital cellulitis, 82
oseltamivir, 47
Osler, William, 6
osteomyelitis, 82
otitis media, *see* earaches
otoscopes, 193
oxygen, 16–17, 19, 46, 111, 116, 128,
    156
    pneumonia and, 131–32, 133, 138,
        139, 144, 147, 148, 168
ozone, 111

pain, 14, 27, 31–35, 141, 183
    chest, 65, 98, 115, 127, 129, 130, 131,
        137, 143, 148, 168, 169, 185, 220,
        229–30
    colds and, 7, 9, 31–34, 64
    in ear, *see* earaches
    around eyes, 65, 66, 82
    influenza and, 4, 31–34, 187
    stomach, 119, 182, 187
Panama H3N3, 163
parainfluenza virus, 61, 184, 195
parapneumonic effusion, 141
Pasteur, Louis, 3
Pauling, Linus, 54
penicillin, 37–38, 150, 207, 223
    allergies to, 38, 39, 80, 124, 183
    for children, 183
    resistance to, 20, 21, 37, 187
    for strep throat, 123, 124, 126
Penny, Carla, 113–14
pens, 7, 63, 70, 81
peptic ulcers, 32, 33

pets, 35–36, 84, 113
phagocytosis, 51
phenol, 35
phenylephrine, 80, 214
phlegm, 102, 106, 113, 115, 135, 173,
    220–21
plaque formation, 22
pleura, *15*, 16, 98, 131
pleurisy, 8, 98–99, 131
Pliny the Elder, 3
pneumonia, 2, 8–9, 16, 65, 117, 127–52,
    202, 213, 231
    bronchial, 9, 128
    causes of, 18–22, 26, 37, 45, 61, 119,
        129
    in children, 67, 130, 145, 177, 184–87
    community-acquired, 128, 129
    deaths from, 2, 8, 45, 67, 128, 139, 169
    hospitalization for, 9, 128, 138–39,
        143, 144, 146–47, 148, 184
    incidence of, 8, 127
    influenza and, 155, 156, 159, 161,
        168–69
    lobar, 9, 128
    mycoplasma, 26, 129, 149–52,
        186–87
    nosocomial, 128–29
    vaccine for, *see* vaccine, for pneumonia
    viral, 129, 145–48, 168, 177, 184–85
pneumonia, bacterial, 18–23, 98, 129–45,
    148
    in children, 177, 185–86
    complications of, 141–42
    diagnosis of, 78, 134–38
    impact of the infection in, 132–34
    prevention of, 45, 142–43, 144,
        171–72, 185–86
    symptoms of, 115, 129–32, 168, 169
    treatment of, 34, 39, 128, 138–41,
        143–44
polio, 23, 24
polymorphonuclear leukocytes (PMN),
    103
polyps, 85–86, 213
Poole, Edna, 138–39
prednisone, 224
pregnancy, 9, 32, 41, 56, 170, 197, 204–7
    antibiotics and, 223–24
premature birth, 191
prostaglandins, 31, 32, 33, 63, 64, 71,
    103, 172
pseudoephedrines, 29, 178, 214
pseudoephrine, 91

Pseudomonas aeruginosa (pseudomonas), 18, 21–22, 136
Pulmicort, 111
pulmonary disease, 134
  see also COPD
pulmonary disorder, *see* lung disease

question-and-answer section, 10, 216–31
quinolones, 39, 79, 92, 204, 207, 224
Qvar, 100, 112

RAT (rapid antigen test), 121
red blood cells, 19, 151
Relenza, 99, 105, 112, 147, 148, 174
  individual needs and, 200, 203
remodeling, 86, 107
Renard, Steven, 48
respirators, 144, 148
respiratory syncytial virus (RSV), 25–26, 61, 145, 184, 190, 191
reverse genetics, influenza and, 164–65
Reye's syndrome, 32, 169, 177–78, 188
rheumatic fever, 20, 118, 119, 122, 125–26, 183
rhinitis, 85
Rhinocort, 90
rhinoviruses, 25, 52, 61, 63, 70, 76
ribavirin, 191
rimantadine, 46–47
Rocephin, 38, 143
Rodriguez, Nancy, 6
Rome, ancient, 3, 23, 54, 55–56

Sacks, Oliver, 155
sailors, 54, 166
salasin, 31
salicylate, 31
saline nasal spray, 81, 181
saline rinses, 49–50, 73, 79, 105, 122, 125, 174, 222
  individual needs and, 207, 212, 215
saliva, 26, 64, 135
SARS (severe adult respiratory syndrome), 2, 61, 62, 218, 224
schools, 117, 122, 123, 186
scurvy, 54, 207
septicemia, 141
Serevent, 112
serology, 149
serotonin inhibitors, 78
Shope, Richard, 156
showers, hot, 49, 73, 81, 92, 101, 103–4, 105, 113, 151, 195, 207, 215, 228

sickle-cell anemia, 41, 46, 188
Singulair, 89, 91
sinus cavities, 13–14, *13*, 74–75, 76, 228
sinuses, 6, 37, 38, 147
sinusitis, 2, 7, 39, 65, 66, 74–93, 213, 217, 231
  causes of, 20, 21, 22, 67, 75–76, 200, 228
  in children, 177, 179–81
  influenza and, 156
sinusitis, acute, 7, 75–84, 179–81
  causes of, 75–76
  complications of, 81–83
  diagnosis of, 77–78
  prevention of, 79, 81, 82
  symptoms of, 75, 78, 85, 86
  treatment of, 78–81, 88–89, 181
sinusitis, chronic, 7, 49–50, 75, 84–93, 179
  complications of, 87–88
  diagnosis of, 86
  impact of infection in, 85–86
  prevention of, 93
  symptoms of, 85
  treatment of, 49–50, 89–92
sinus X-rays, 65, 77, 78, 86
skin, 19, 24
sleep, 28, 29, 72, 157, 176, 226
smallpox, 5, 23, 44, 45
smell, sense of, 13, 227, 231
smoking, smoke, 17, 167, 210
  bronchitis and, 94, 96, 102, 106–9, 168, 181, 231
  cilia and, 14, 85, 106, 140, 227
  colds and, 6, 69, 157, 227–28, 230, 231
  coughs and, 35–36
  pneumonia and, 130, 134, 140–41, 231
  secondhand, 107, 113, 181, 192, 193, 208, 213
smooth muscles, 17, 29, 30, 36
  bronchitis and, 94, *95*
sneezing, 2, 5, 11, 28, 60, 63, 64, 66, 68, 130, 187, 218, 220
  influenza and, 156, 157, 173
  treatment for, 28, 173
soap, 70
soda, 202
  diet, 47, 73, 92, 105
sore throats, 2, 6, 8, 15, 28, 60, 117–18, 168
  in children, 176, 182, 186

treatment for, 48, 49, 50, 56, 73, 117, 118–19, 172, 173, 222, 224, 225, 226
see also strep throat
soups, 103, 105, 181
vegetable, 201, 227
see also chicken soup
Spanish flu (1918), 4–5, 23, 24, 154–55, 160, 167
sphenoid sinus, *13*, 75
spicy foods, 48–49, 81, 101, 105, 125
spinal cord, *13*, 82
spinal tap, 83
Spiriva, 111, 112
spirometry, 97, 108, 115
Staphylococcus aureus (staph), 19–20, 103
steroids, 90, 91, 142, 151, 172, 180
bronchitis and, 111, 112, 116
stomach, 32, 88, 155
mucus in, 12–13, 14
pain in, 119, 182, 187
vitamin C and, 55, 227
Stone, Rev. Edmund, 31
strep throat, 8, 18, 117–26
antibiotics for, 8, 39, 117, 118, 123, 124
causes of, 18, 20, 37, 119
in children, 117, 122, 123, 126, 182–84
complications of, 118, 119, 125–26, 183
diagnosis of, 78, 120–22, 220
prevention of, 123, 205
symptoms of, 119–20, 182
transmission of, 122–23
treatment for, 8, 39, 117, 118, 122–25, 183–84
streptococcus bacteria, 45, 76, 103, 118–22, 171
Streptococcus pneumoniae (pneumococcus), 20, 22, 129, 136, 142, 144, 185, 192
Streptococcus pyogenes (strep), 20, 136
streptokinase, 120
streptolysin, 120
stress, 4, 229
sulfa drugs, allergies to, 80
supplements, 51–56, 73
individual needs and, 200, 204, 206–7, 209–10, 212, 215
surgery, 141, 183–84, 223
sinus, 7, 90, 181
for sinusitis complications, 82, 83

swelling, 27, 64, 82, 90, 145, 183
bronchitis and, 94, *95*, 103
in glands, 119, 124, 176, 182
swine flu, 43, 159, 162, 163, 171

Tamiflu, 47, 99, 101, 105, 112, 147, 148, 157, 172, 173, 188
individual needs and, 200, 203, 209, 214–15
taste, sense of, 227, 231
tea, 47, 51, 73, 215
elderberry, *55*–56
green, 227
hot, 48, 71–72, 73, 81, 92, 101, 103, 105, 125, 151, 174, 182, 207, 215, 226, 229
iced, 73, 125, 174
telephones, 26, 63, 79, 219
temperature, 221–22, 229–30
see also fever
Tequin, 39, 150, 204
tetracyclines, 151, 187, 207, 223–24
theobromines, 48, 227
theophylline, 111, 112
thimerosal, 44, 188
Third National Health and Nutrition Examination Survey (NHANESIII), 109
throat, 6, 12–16, *13*, 19, 24, 28, 37, 157, 167
mucus in, 12, 14, 84
sore, *see* sore throats; strep throats
see also coughs
throat cultures, 8, 120–22, 183, 220
tissues, 63, 70
tonsillitis, 8, 223
tonsils, *13*, 14–15, 119, 120, 124, 182, 183–84, 223
Toronto study, 69–70
trachea, *13*, *15*, 16, 84, 96, 166, 168
transillumination, 77, 180
treatment, 7, 9, 27–58, 221–27
see also decongestants; hydrotherapy; nutritional therapy; vaccines; *specific drugs*; *specific respiratory infections*
trivalent inactivated influenza virus, 40
turbinates, 12, *13*
Tylenol, 32–33, 35, 71
individual needs and, 199, 205, 209
Tylenol Cold Day Non-Drowsy, 29

urinary tract infections, 21, 39, 136, 202

vaccine, influenza, 5, 9, 39–45, 153,
    162–65, 174
    bacterial contamination of, 41, 42
    bronchitis and, 96, 99, 101, 105, 112,
        115
    children and, 185, 188–89, 193, 196
    effectiveness of, 67, 162–63, 200, 214,
        217–18
    pneumonia and, 144, 146, 147
    production of, 42–45
    public resistance to, 42, 162–63
    shortage of, 42–45, 170, 198
    types of, 40
    who should get, 41, 169–71, 200, 203,
        206, 209, 211, 214
vaccines, 24, 39–46, 80, 191
    for children, 41, 44, 67, 169–72,
        185–86, 188–89, 191, 192, 193,
        195, 196
    colds and, 39, 73
    Hib, 195, 196
    individual needs and, 200, 203, 206,
        209, 211, 214
    lawsuits and, 43–44
    for meningitis, 21, 43
    for pneumonia, 12, 39, 43, 45–46, 112,
        115, 127, 142–43, 144, 171–72,
        174, 185–86, 196, 200, 203, 211
    smallpox, 44, 45
Ventolin HFA, 36
Vicks Formula 44, 35
viruses, 6, 11–14, 17, 18, 23–26, 219
    antibiotics and, 11, 36
    bacteria compared with, 24, 120
    bronchitis and, see bronchitis, acute
        viral
    cold, 4, 7, 11, 13, 25, 28, 29, 60–64,
        68, 76, 145, 157–58, 217
    croup and, 195
    influenza, 4, 9, 21, 24, 25, 28, 67, 145,
        153–72, 161, 195
    mycoplasma compared with, 26
    pneumonia and, 129, 145–48, 168,
        177, 184–85
    replication of, 7, 24, 25, 63, 81, 145,
        224
    sinusitis and, 75, 77, 78

    sore throats and, 8, 117
    surveillance of, 5
    see also antibodies
vision, double, 82, 83
vitamin A, 55, 109, 206–7, 210
vitamin C, 54–55, 73, 109, 221, 227
    individual needs and, 200, 204, 207,
        210, 212, 215
vitamin D, 206–7
vitamin E, 55, 109, 210, 215
voice, loss of, 15, 60, 194
vomiting, 182, 187, 202

water, 22
    drinking of, 47, 73, 92, 105, 207, 215
    see also hydrotherapy
whiskey cure, 6–7
white blood cells, 14, 18, 20, 21, 48, 51,
        64, 115, 141
    death of, 102–3
    increase in, 83, 103
    pneumonia and, 131, 134, 142
    streptococcus and, 120
willow, 31
wine, as cold remedy, 3
World Health Organization (WHO), 36,
        40, 160
World War I, 23, 24, 155
World War II, 156
Wyeth pharmaceuticals, 43
Wyle, Thomas, 4

X-rays:
    chest, see chest X-rays
    sinus, 65, 77, 78, 86

zanamivir (Relenza), 47
Ziment, Irwin, 48–49
zinc, 52–54, 73
    individual needs and, 200, 204, 212,
        215
zinc acetate, 53
zinc gluconate, 53, 81
zinc lozenges, 53, 73, 200, 204
zinc nasal spray, 53, 81, 82
zinc pills, 53–54
Zithromax, 39, 124, 151, 173